# Cancer-related Breakthrough Pain

O P M L

OXFORD PAIN MANAGEMENT LIBRARY

# Cancer-related Breakthrough Pain

Editor

## Dr Andrew Davies

Consultant in Palliative Medicine,
The Royal Marsden Hospital,
Sutton, UK

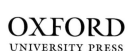

OXFORD
UNIVERSITY PRESS

# OXFORD
UNIVERSITY PRESS

Great Clarendon Street, Oxford OX2 6DP

Oxford University Press is a department of the University of Oxford.
It furthers the University's objective of excellence in research, scholarship,
and education by publishing worldwide in

Oxford New York

Auckland Cape Town Dar es Salaam Hong Kong Karachi
Kuala Lumpur Madrid Melbourne Mexico City Nairobi
New Delhi Shanghai Taipei Toronto

With offices in

Argentina Austria Brazil Chile Czech Republic France Greece
Guatemala Hungary Italy Japan Poland Portugal Singapore
South Korea Switzerland Thailand Turkey Ukraine Vietnam

Oxford is a registered trade mark of Oxford University Press
in the UK and in certain other countries

Published in the United States
by Oxford University Press Inc., New York

British Library Cataloguing in Publication Data

Data available

Library of Congress Cataloging in Publication Data

Data available

Typeset by Newgen Imaging Systems (P) Ltd, Chennai, India
Printed in the United Kingdom
on acid-free paper by CPI Bath Press

ISBN 0–19–921567–7 978–0–19–921567–6

10 9 8 7 6 5 4 3 2 1

# Contents

# Contributors

**Andrew Davies**
Consultant in Palliative Medicine
The Royal Marsden Hospital,
Sutton, United Kingdom
*Chapter 1 Introduction*
*Chapter 2 Clinical features*
*Chapter 3 Assessment*
*Chapter 4 General principles of
management*
*Chapter 8 Non-opioid drugs*

**Fiona Bailey**
Specialist Registrar in
Palliative Medicine
St. Christopher's Hospice,
London, United Kingdom
*Chapter 5 Oral opioid drugs*

**Nicholas Christelis**
Locum Consultant in
Anaesthesia
Chelsea & Westminster Hospital,
London, United Kingdom
*Chapter 9 Other therapeutic
interventions*

**Ola Dale**
Professor of Anesthesiology/
Pharmacology
Norwegian University of Science
and Technology,
Trondheim, Norway
*Chapter 7 Opioid drugs via other
routes*

**Ann Farley**
Specialist Sister in
Palliative Care
The Royal Marsden Hospital,
Sutton, United Kingdom
*Chapter 5 Oral opioid drugs*

**Jackie Filshie**
Consultant in Anaesthesia and
Pain Management
The Royal Marsden Hospital,
Sutton, United Kingdom
*Chapter 9 Other therapeutic
interventions*

**Craig Gannon**
Consultant in Palliative Medicine
Princess Alice Hospice, Esher,
United Kingdom
*Chapter 8 Non-opioid drugs*

**Diane Laverty**
Lead Nurse Bereavement
Services
Royal Free Hospital, London,
United Kingdom
*Chapter 3 Assessment*

**Charles Skinner**
Specialist Registrar in Palliative
Medicine
The Royal Marsden Hospital,
Sutton, United Kingdom
*Chapter 2 Clinical features*

**Emma Thompson**
Specialist Registrar in Palliative
Medicine
The Royal Marsden Hospital,
Sutton, United Kingdom
*Chapter 2 Clinical features*

**Giovambattista
Zeppetella**
Consultant in Palliative Medicine
St. Clare Hospice,
Hastingwood, United Kingdom
*Chapter 6 Oral transmucosal
opioid drugs*

# Chapter 1

# Introduction

Andrew Davies

*'You can't find it [inner peace] in that darkness of pain ... I can't
emphasize that the pain blinds you to all of that, blinds you to all
that's positive. I mean the real bad pain ... it just closes you
down. You just can't get through it ... it's an iron door and it's one
thing you don't wanna go through ... you just wanna, wanna stop'*
(Coyle 2004)

## 1.1 **Introduction**

Over the last 15 years, there has been an increasing interest in the
phenomenon of breakthrough pain. This upsurge in interest has been
generated by a greater awareness of the problem of breakthrough pain
(secondary to improvements in the management of background pain),
and has been fuelled by an increasing range of pharmacological options
for the treatment of breakthrough pain (Colleau 1999).

The focus of this book is on cancer-related breakthrough pain.
However, breakthrough pain may also occur in patients with
non-malignant diseases. Thus, Zeppetella et al reported that breakthrough pain was very common in patients with non-malignant
diseases admitted to a hospice in the United Kingdom (i.e. 63% of
patients that reported background pain) (Zeppetella et al 2001).

## 1.2 **Definitions**

• Pain
The standard definition of pain is 'an unpleasant sensory and emo-
tional experience associated with actual or potential tissue damage,
or described in terms of such damage' (Anonymous 1994).

• Background pain
Background pain refers to 'constant or continuous pain of long duration' (Ferrell et al 1999). It should be noted that the phrase 'long
duration' refers to a period of ≥12 hr/day (Ferrell et al 1999).

The term background pain is widely used in the United Kingdom.
However, other terms are used in the medical literature to describe
the same phenomenon, including 'basal pain', 'baseline pain', and
'persistent pain' (Ferrell et al 1999).

### Fig 1.1 Definitions of breakthrough pain

- 'A transitory exacerbation of pain that occurs on a background of otherwise stable pain in a patient receiving chronic opioid therapy' (Portenoy & Hagen, 1990).
- 'A transitory increase in pain to greater than moderate intensity (that is, to an intensity of 'severe' or 'excruciating'), which occurred on a baseline pain of moderate intensity or less (that is, no pain or pain of 'mild' or 'moderate' intensity) (Portenoy & Hagen 1990).
- 'A transitory exacerbation of pain experienced by the patient who has relatively stable and adequately controlled baseline pain' (Portenoy et al 2004).

- Breakthrough pain

A recent definition of breakthrough pain is 'a transitory exacerbation of pain experienced by the patient who has relatively stable and adequately controlled baseline pain' (Portenoy et al 2004). Figure 1.1 shows some of the earlier definitions of breakthrough pain (Portenoy & Hagen 1990).

The term breakthrough pain is widely used. However, other terms are also used in the medical literature to describe the same phenomenon, including 'episodic pain', 'exacerbation of pain', 'pain flare', 'transient pain', and 'transitory pain' (Colleau 1999).

'Breakthrough pain' is an English term; an equivalent term does not exist in certain European languages (e.g. French, Italian, Spanish) (Colleau 1999). On the basis of this fact, an Expert Working Group of the European Association for Palliative Care (EAPC) has suggested that the term 'breakthrough pain' should be replaced by the terms 'episodic pain' or 'transient pain' (Mercadante et al 2002). However, the term 'breakthrough pain' is still widely used in the medical literature, and still used by members of the Expert Working Group of the EAPC (Caraceni et al 2004).

## 1.3 Classifications

Breakthrough pain can be classified according to its relationship to specific events, or to analgesic dosing (Davies 2005):

- Spontaneous pain (also known as 'idiopathic pain') – this type of pain occurs unexpectedly.
- Incident pain (also known as 'precipitated pain' or, when appropriate, 'movement-related pain') – this type of pain is related to specific events, and can be subclassified into three categories:
  1. Volitional – pain is precipitated by a voluntary act (e.g. walking).
  2. Non-volitional – pain is precipitated by an involuntary act (e.g. coughing).
  3. Procedural – this type of pain is related to a therapeutic intervention (e.g. wound dressing).

- End-of-dose failure – this type of pain is related to analgesic dosing (i.e. declining analgesic levels).

As discussed above, the diagnosis of breakthrough pain relies on the co-existence of 'adequately controlled background pain' (Portenoy et al 2004). Some authors do not regard end-of-dose failure as a subtype of breakthrough pain, since they perceive that end-of-dose failure represents inadequately controlled background pain (Simmonds 1999); nevertheless, most authors do regard end-of-dose failure as a subtype of breakthrough pain (assuming the co-existence of adequately controlled breakthrough pain for a period of over half of the time). Table 1.2 shows the prevalence of breakthrough pain subtypes in studies published in English and applying standard criteria for breakthrough pain (Fine & Busch 1998; Gómez-Batiste et al 2002; Hwang et al 2003; Portenoy & Hagen 1990; Portenoy et al 1999; Zeppetella et al 2000).

## 1.4 Epidemiology

Pain is a common problem in patients with cancer. Indeed, the prevalence of pain has been reported to be 30–40% amongst patients with early disease (receiving anti-cancer therapy), and 70–90% amongst patients with advanced disease (Foley 2004).

Similarly, breakthrough pain is a common problem in patients with cancer. The prevalence of breakthrough pain has been reported to be 19–95% amongst various groups of patients (Zeppetella & Ribeiro 2003). This disparity reflects a number of factors, including differences in the definition applied (see below), methods utilized, and in population studied (Mercadante et al 2002). Furthermore, the reporting of breakthrough pain is affected by certain language/geographical variables (see below).

Many authors have adopted the diagnostic criteria for breakthrough pain employed by Portenoy & Hagen (1990). These criteria are:

1) the presence of stable analgesia in the previous 48 hr
2) the presence of controlled background pain in the previous 24 hr (i.e. average pain intensity of none, mild or moderate for over half of the previous 24 hr)
3) the presence of 'temporary flares of severe or excruciating pain' in the previous 24 hr.

Table 1.1 shows the prevalence of breakthrough pain in studies published in English and applying standard criteria for breakthrough pain (Fine & Busch 1998; Fortner et al 2002; Fortner et al 2003; Gomez-Batiste et al 2002; Hwang et al 2003; Portenoy & Hagen 1990; Portenoy et al 1999; Zeppetella et al 2000). It should be noted that these figures represent the prevalence of breakthrough pain in selected populations of cancer patients, rather than the prevalence of breakthrough pain in the general population of cancer patients.

**Table 1.1** Prevalence of breakthrough pain in studies applying standard criteria for breakthrough pain

| Study | Population | Prevalence of breakthrough pain | Comments |
|---|---|---|---|
| Portenoy & Hagen (1990) | Hospital inpatients (pain-team referrals) – USA n = 90 | 63% | Criteria for BTP outlined in this study. 90 patients assessed; 63 patients reported controlled background pain; 41 patients reported BTP. |
| Fine & Busch (1998) | Palliative care patients (home setting) – USA n = 22 | 86% | Only patients with pain eligible. 22 patients assessed; 22 patients reported background pain; 19 patients reported BTP. |
| Portenoy et al (1999) | Hospital inpatients – USA n = 178 | 51% | Only patients on regular opioid analgesics eligible. 178 patients assessed; 164 patients reported controlled background pain; 84 patients reported BTP. |
| Zeppetella et al (2000) | Hospice inpatients – UK n = 414 | 89% | 381 patients assessed (33 patients not assessable); 245 patients reported background pain; 218 patients reported BTP. |

| | | |
|---|---|---|
| Fortner et al (2002) | Cancer patients (home setting) – USA n = 1000 | 63% | Telephone survey of cancer patients. 1000 patients assessed; 256 patients reported regular analgesic usage; 160 patients reported BTP. |
| Gómez-Batiste et al (2002) | Palliative care patients (various settings) – Spain n = 407 | 41% | 397 patients assessed (10 patients not assessable); 163 patients reported BTP. |
| Fortner et al (2003) | Cancer patients (outpatient setting) – USA n = 373 | 23% | Non-specific data relating to the patients' pain scores/pain medications were used to diagnose presence of BTP. 373 patients assessed; 144 patients reported background pain; 33 patients were deemed to have BTP. |
| Hwang et al (2003) | VA hospital patients (in/outpatient setting) – USA n = 74 | 70% | Only patients with pain eligible. 74 patients assessed, 74 patients reported background pain; 52 patients reported BTP. After a week of treatment, BTP prevalence decreased from 70% to 36%. |

BTP = breakthrough pain; VA = Veterans Affairs.

Interestingly, the International Association for the Study of Pain (IASP) survey of cancer pain characteristics and syndromes found that pain specialists from English-speaking (North America, Australasia) and Northern/Western European countries reported more breakthrough pain than pain specialists from South American, Asian, and Southern/Eastern European countries (Caraceni & Portenoy 1999; Caraceni et al 2004).

Breakthrough pain appears to be more common in patients with advanced disease (Colleau 2004), in patients with poor performance status (Caraceni et al 2004), in patients with pain originating from the vertebral column (and to a lesser extent other weight-bearing bones/joints) (Caraceni et al 2004) and in patients with pain originating from the nerve plexuses (and to a lesser extent nerve roots) (Caraceni et al 2004).

## 1.5 Aetiology

The aetiology of the breakthrough pain is often the same as that of the background pain (Portenoy & Hagen 1990; Portenoy et al 1999). Thus, breakthrough pain may be due to (Zeppetella & Ribeiro 2003):

a) direct effect of the cancer

b) indirect effect of the cancer (i.e. secondary to disability)

c) anti-cancer treatment

d) concomitant illness.

Indeed, breakthrough pain may be experienced by patients at all stages of cancer (at diagnosis, during active treatment, during remission, during relapse/progression, following cure) (Portenoy & Hagen 1990; Portenoy et al 1999). Table 1.3 shows the aetiology of breakthrough pain in relevant published studies (Portenoy & Hagen 1990; Portenoy et al 1999; Zeppetella et al 2000).

Not surprisingly, the pathophysiology of the breakthrough pain is also often the same as that of the background pain. Thus breakthrough pain may be: a) nociceptive; b) neuropathic; or c) mixed (nociceptive and neuropathic). Table 1.3 shows the pathophysiology of breakthrough pain in relevant published studies (Portenoy & Hagen, 1990, Portenoy et al, 1999; Zeppetella et al, 2000).

**Table 1.2 Prevalence of breakthrough pain subtypes in studies using standard criteria for breakthrough pain**

| Study | Prevalence of breakthrough pain subtypes | | | Comments |
|---|---|---|---|---|
| | Spontaneous pain | Incident pain | End-of-dose failure | |
| Portenoy & Hagen (1990) | 27% | 43% | 18% | 12% of pain reports were 'mixed' in nature (incident and end-of-dose failure). Incident pain precipitants: movement 22%; coughing 12%; sitting 4%; touch 2%. |
| Fine & Busch (1998) | No data | ~50% | No data | No further details in paper. |
| Portenoy et al (1999) | 38% | 49% | 13% | Incident pain precipitants: movement 27.8%; defaecation 5.7%; urination 3.8%; coughing 3.7%; sitting 3.7%; breathing 1.9%; eating/drinking 1.9%. |
| Zeppetella et al (2000) | 59% | 24% | 17% | No further details in paper. |
| Gómez-Batiste et al (2002) | 32% | 52% | 15% | Incident pain precipitants: movement 38%; eating/drinking 3%; defaecation 2%; coughing 2%. |
| Hwang et al (2003) | 17% | 64% | 19% | Data based on initial assessment of patient. Incident precipitants: movement 44%; coughing 4%; eating/drinking 4%; defaecation 2%; sitting 2%. |

**Table 1.3 Aetiology and pathophysiology of breakthrough pain**

| Study | Aetiology | | | Pathophysiology | | |
|---|---|---|---|---|---|---|
| | Cancer | Cancer treatment | Concomitant disease | Nociceptive pain | Neuropathic pain | Mixed pain |
| Portenoy & Hagen (1990) | 76% | 20% | 4% | 53% | 27% | 20% |
| Portenoy et al (1999) | 65% | 35% | 0% | 38% | 10% | 52% |
| Zeppetella et al (2000) | 71% | 11% | 19% | 74% | 9% | 16% |

## 1.6 Clinical features

Breakthrough pain is not a single entity, but a spectrum of very different entities. The clinical features vary from individual to individual and may vary within an individual over time (Portenoy 1997). However, the clinical features of the breakthrough pain are often related to the clinical features of the background pain (Portenoy et al 1999).

There appears to be an association between the presence of breakthrough pain and the intensity/frequency of the background pain (i.e. patients with breakthrough pain often have more severe/more frequent background pain) (Caraceni et al 2004; Portenoy et al 1999). Indeed, breakthrough pain is associated with poor overall pain control (Bruera et al 1995; Mercadante et al 1992) and, not surprisingly, decreased satisfaction with overall pain control (Zeppetella et al 2000).

Breakthrough pain may result in a number of other physical, psychological, and social problems (see Chapter 2). Indeed, breakthrough pain has a significant negative impact on quality of life (Hwang et al 2003; Portenoy et al 1999). The degree of interference seems to be related to the characteristics of the breakthrough pain: patients with spontaneous pain (Portenoy et al 1999) and patients with severe pain (Swanwick et al 2000) may experience particular problems.

Not surprisingly breakthrough pain is associated with increased use of healthcare services (i.e. increased outpatient visits, increased inpatient admissions) (Fortner et al 2002). This results in an increase in direct costs (e.g. prescription costs), and in indirect costs (e.g. transportation costs) for both the health service, the patient, and their carers (Fortner et al 2003).

## 1.7 Conclusions

The preceding quotation exemplifies the negative effects of poorly controlled cancer pain (Coyle 2004), whilst the subsequent quotation (from the same patient) reinforces the positive effects of well controlled cancer pain (Coyle 2004). Breakthrough pain is a major challenge to healthcare professionals (as well as to their patients). Nevertheless, in many cases, it is possible to eradicate the breakthrough pain (Hwang et al 2003). Moreover, in all cases, it should be possible to ameliorate the breakthrough pain. The following chapters will address the issues of the assessment, the general principles of management, and the specific options for management of cancer-related breakthrough pain.

> 'Once the pain was relieved it was the most beautiful experience of my life, to be able to participate and control the pain'

> (Coyle 2004)

# References

Anonymous (1994). In Merskey, H., Bogduk, N., ed. *Classification of Chronic Pain* (2nd edn). IASP Press, Seattle, 209–214.

Bruera, E., Schoeller, T., Wenk, R., *et al.* (1995). A prospective multicenter assessment of the Edmonton Staging System for cancer pain. *Journal of Pain and Symptom Management*, **10**: 348–355.

Caraceni, A., Portenoy, R.K. (1999). An international survey of cancer pain characteristics and syndromes. *Pain*, **82**: 263–274.

Caraceni, A., Martini, C., Zecca, E., *et al.* (2004). Breakthrough pain characteristics and syndromes in patients with cancer pain. An international survey. *Palliative Medicine*, **18**: 177–183.

Coyle, N. (2004). In their own words: seven advanced cancer patients describe their experience with pain and the use of opioid drugs. *Journal of Pain and Symptom Management*, **27**: 300–309.

Colleau, S.M. (1999). The significance of breakthrough pain in cancer. *Cancer Pain Release*, **12**: 1–4.

Colleau, S.M. (2004). Breakthrough (episodic) vs. baseline (persistent) pain in cancer. *Cancer Pain Release*, **17**: 1–3.

Davies, A. (2005). Current thinking in cancer breakthrough pain management. *European Journal of Palliative Care*, **12** (Suppl): 4–6.

Ferrell, B.R., Juarez, G., Borneman, T. (1999). Use of routine and breakthrough analgesia in home care. *Oncology Nursing Forum*, **26**: 1655–1661.

Fine, P.G., Busch, M.A. (1998). Characterization of breakthrough pain by hospice patients and their caregivers. *Journal of Pain and Symptom Management*, **16**: 179–183.

Foley, K.M. (2004). Acute and chronic cancer pain syndromes. In Doyle, D., Hanks, G., Cherny, N., Calman, K., ed. *Oxford Textbook of Palliative Medicine* (3rd edn). Oxford University Press, Oxford, 298–316.

Fortner, B.V., Okon, T.A., Portenoy, R. K. (2002). A survey of pain-related hospitalizations, emergency department visits, and physician office visits reported by cancer patients with and without history of breakthrough pain. *Journal of Pain*, **3**: 38–44.

Fortner, B.V., Demarco, G., Irving, G., *et al.* (2003). Description and predictors of direct and indirect costs of pain reported by cancer patients. *Journal of Pain and Symptom Management*, **25**: 9–18.

Gómez-Batiste, X., Madrid, F., Moreno, F., *et al.* (2002). Breakthrough cancer pain: prevalence and characteristics in patients in Catalonia, Spain. *Journal of Pain and Symptom Management*, **24**: 45–52.

Hwang, S.S., Chang, V.T., Kasimis, B. (2003). Cancer breakthrough pain characteristics and responses to treatment at a VA medical center. *Pain*, **101**: 55–64.

Mercadante, S., Maddaloni, S., Roccella, S., Salvaggio, L. (1992). Predictive factors in advanced cancer pain treated only by analgesics. *Pain*, **50**: 151–155.

Mercadante, S., Radbruch, L., Caraceni, A., et al. (2002). Episodic (break-through) pain. Consensus Conference of an Expert Working Group of the European Association for Palliative Care. *Cancer*, **94**: 832–839.

Portenoy, R.K., Hagen, N.A. (1990). Breakthrough pain: definition, preva-lence and characteristics. *Pain*, **41**: 273–281.

Portenoy, R.K. (1997). Treatment of temporal variations in chronic cancer pain. *Seminars in Oncology*, **5**: (Suppl 16): S16–7–12.

Portenoy, R.K., Payne, D., Jacobsen, P. (1999). Breakthrough pain: charac-teristics and impact in patients with cancer pain. *Pain*, **81**: 129–134.

Portenoy, R.K., Forbes, K., Lussier, D., Hanks, G. (2004). Difficult pain problems: an integrated approach. In Doyle D., Hanks G., Cherny N., Calman K., ed. *Oxford Textbook of Palliative Medicine* (3rd edn). Oxford University Press, Oxford, 438–458.

Simmonds, M.A. (1999). Management of breakthrough pain due to cancer. *Oncology (Huntington)*, **13**: 1103–1108.

Swanwick, M., Haworth, M., Lennard, R.F. (2001). The prevalence of episodic pain in cancer: a survey of hospice patients on admission. *Palliative Medicine*, **15**: 9–18.

Zeppetella, G., O'Doherty, C.A., Collins, S., (2000). Prevalence and characteristics of breakthrough pain in cancer patients admitted to a hospice. *Journal of Pain and Symptom Management*, **20**: 87–92.

Zeppetella, G., O'Doherty, C.A., Collins, S. (2001). Prevalence and char-acteristics of breakthrough pain in patients with non-malignant terminal disease admitted to a hospice. *Palliative Medicine*, **15**: 243–246.

Zeppetella, G., Ribeiro, M.D. (2003). Pharmacotherapy of cancer-related episodic pain. *Expert Opinion on Pharmacotherapy*, **4**: 493–502.

# Chapter 2

# Clinical features

Charles Skinner, Emma Thompson &
Andrew Davies

## 2.1 Introduction

Breakthrough pain has been defined as 'a transitory exacerbation of pain experienced by the patient who has relatively stable and adequately controlled baseline pain' (Portenoy et al 2004). This definition is very broad and reflects the fact that breakthrough pain is very diverse in nature. Thus, breakthrough pain can have multiple causes with multiple pathophysiologies, and can present with numerous clinical features and numerous complications. In some cases, breakthrough pain is a mere inconvenience, but in many cases breakthrough pain is a cause of significant morbidity.

## 2.2 Classification

As discussed in Chapter 1, breakthrough pain can be classified according to its relationship to specific events or to analgesic dosing (Davies 2005):

- Spontaneous pain (also known as 'idiopathic pain') – this type of pain occurs unexpectedly.
- Incident pain (also known as 'precipitated pain' or, when appropriate, 'movement-related pain') – this type of pain is related to specific events, and can be subclassified into three categories:
  - Volitional – pain is precipitated by a voluntary act (e.g. walking).
  - Non-volitional – pain is precipitated by an involuntary act (e.g. coughing).
  - Procedural – pain is related to a therapeutic intervention (e.g. wound dressing).
- End-of-dose failure – this type of pain is related to analgesic dosing, i.e. declining analgesic levels. (It should be noted that some authors do not regard end-of-dose failure as a subtype of breakthrough pain (Simmonds 1999)).

Table 1.2 shows the breakdown of the different types of breakthrough pain in studies that have applied standard criteria for diagnosing breakthrough pain (Fine & Busch 1998; Gómez-Batiste et al 2002;

Hwang *et al* 2003; Portenoy & Hagen 1990; Portenoy *et al* 1999; Zeppetella *et al* 2000). Figures 2.1–2.3 illustrate case histories from patients with the different types of breakthrough pain.

### Fig 2.1a  Case history of a patient with spontaneous-type breakthrough pain

Mr PW was a 50-year-old man with localized Ewing's sarcoma of the sacrum (Figure 2.1b). He presented to the palliative care team with severe pain in the penis/scrotum secondary to the primary tumour. This pain was intermittent in nature occurring 3–4 times per hour and lasting <1 min per episode. (There were no precipitating/aggravating factors). He also complained of moderate pain in the gluteal area/legs secondary to the primary tumour. This pain was persistent in nature. The patient had been receiving paracetamol and low doses of gabapentin for the pain.

The paracetamol was replaced by cocodamol 30/500, which resulted in good control of the persistent pain (The cocodamol 30/500 had no effect on the spontaneous pain). In addition, the gabapentin was titrated upwards, which resulted in good control of the spontaneous pain. During this period the patient also received an epidural injection of steroid (which had little effect on the pain) and a course of radical radiotherapy to the sacrum (which initially aggravated the pain). In due course, following completion of his multimodal oncological therapy, the patient was able to discontinue all of the aforementioned analgesics.

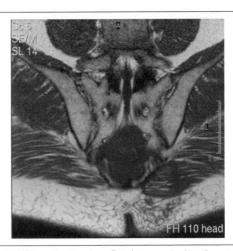

**Figure 2.1b**  MRI scan showing primary Ewing's sarcoma involving the sacrum (in a patient with spontaneous pain)

## Fig 2.2a Case history of a patient with incident-type breakthrough pain

Mr ML was a 64-year-old man with advanced renal cell carcinoma. He had widespread bone metastases, including disease in the thoracic spine, lumbar spine and pelvis (particularly the left acetabulum: Figure 2.2b). He complained of pains in the lower back and hip which were present at rest, but more severe on movement. As a result of the incident pain, he was rendered bed bound. Moreover, movement in the bed also resulted in significant pain.

He was started on normal-release morphine sulphate, and the dose was gradually titrated upwards in an attempt to control the pain. The pain at rest was well controlled, but the pain on movement remained uncontrolled, and further titration of the morphine resulted in the development of opioid toxicity. The morphine was switched to oxycodone, but although the opioid toxicity settled, the pain on movement remained uncontrolled.

An epidural catheter was inserted, and an infusion of fentanyl and bupivacaine commenced. This resulted in excellent pain relief, so much so that the patient was able to get out of bed and sit in a chair. Subsequently, following a course of palliative radiotherapy to the lumbar spine, the epidural was able to be removed and conventional analgesics reinstated with continued good pain control (paracetamol, oxycodone).

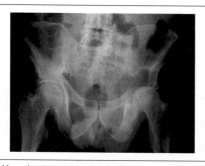

**Figure 2.2b** X-ray showing metastatic renal cell carcinoma involving the acetabulum (in a patient with incident pain)

Breakthrough pain can also be classified according to the underlying pathophysiology of the pain:

- Nociceptive pain – this type of pain is related to stimulation of the nerve endings, and can be subclassified into two categories
  - Somatic pain – pain originates from the cutaneous/ musculoskeletal tissues of the body.
  - Visceral pain – pain originates from the organs of the body.
- Neuropathic pain – this type of pain is related to damage to the nerve structure.
- Mixed pain – a combination of nociceptive and neuropathic pain.

## Fig 2.3  Case history of a patient with end-of-dose failure

Mr LS was a 70-year-old man with metastatic carcinoma of the rectum. He presented to the palliative care team with severe pain in the lumbar spine/rectum secondary to a pelvic recurrence of the tumour. The pain was persistent in nature but was aggravated by walking and sitting down. The patient had been receiving moderate doses of controlled-release morphine for the pain.

The patient was converted to normal-release morphine sulphate, and the dose titrated upwards. The increased dose produced good analgesia but was associated with opioid toxicity. An opioid rotation was performed, with normal-release oxycodone being substituted for the morphine. The oxycodone again produced good analgesia but was associated with auditory hallucinations. Thus, a further opioid rotation was performed with transdermal fentanyl substituted for the oxycodone.

The transdermal fentanyl resulted in good pain control, although the patient reported a significant deterioration in pain control during the hours before the patch was due to be replaced. The dose of transdermal fentanyl was titrated upwards, but this led to the development of confusion. Consequently, the dose of transdermal fentanyl was titrated downwards and the patch was replaced every 48 hr rather than every 72 hr. These changes resulted in the resolution of the confusion and the end-of-dose failure.

16

See Table 1.3 in the previous chapter for the pathophysiologies of breakthrough pain in studies that have applied standard criteria for diagnosing breakthrough pain (Portenoy & Hagen 1990; Portenoy et al 1999; Zeppetella et al 2000).

## 2.3  General features

Breakthrough pain is not a single entity, but a spectrum of very different entities. The clinical features vary from individual to individual, and may vary within an individual over time (Portenoy 1997). However the clinical features of the breakthrough pain are often related to the clinical features of the background pain (Portenoy et al 1999). Table 2.1 shows some of the characteristics of breakthrough pain in studies published in English that have applied standard criteria for diagnosing breakthrough pain (Fine & Busch 1998; Gómez-Batiste et al 2002; Hwang et al 2003; Portenoy & Hagen 1990; Portenoy et al 1999; Zeppetella et al 2000].

The diagnosis of breakthrough pain depends on the presence of well-controlled background pain, and so the initial presentation of breakthrough pain often coincides with the successful management of the background pain. The development/progression of breakthrough pain may signify the progression of underlying pathology, or the development of new pathology (e.g. pathological fracture) (Patt & Ellison 1998). However, the development/progression of breakthrough pain

**Table 2.1a** Characteristics of breakthrough pain in studies applying standard criteria for diagnosis

| Study | BTP connected to background pain | BTP number of sites | Episodes of BTP (episodes/day) | Comments |
|---|---|---|---|---|
| Portenoy & Hagen (1990) | 96% | 1 pain – 78%<br>2 pains – 20%<br>3 pains – 2% | Median 4<br>(range 1–3600) | The patient with 3600 episodes/day had a rib fracture and a persistent cough. |
| Fine & Busch (1998) | – | – | Mean 2.9<br>(range 1–5.5) | |
| Portenoy et al (1999) | 100% | 1 pain – 83.1%<br>2 pains – 14.5%<br>3 pains – 2.4% | Median 6<br>(range 1–60) | |
| Zeppetella et al (2000) | 89% | Mean 2 pains<br>(range 1–5) | Mean 4<br>(range 1–14) | |
| Gómez-Batiste et al (2002) | – | – | Mean 1.5<br>(range 0–5) | |
| Hwang et al (2003) | 75% | 1 pain – 79%<br>≥2 pains – 21% | Median 5<br>(range 1–50) | Data based on initial assessment of patients. |

BTP = breakthrough pain

Table 2.1b **Characteristics of breakthrough pain in studies applying standard criteria for diagnosis**

| Study | Duration BTP (min) | Onset of BTP | Intensity of BTP | Comments |
|---|---|---|---|---|
| Portenoy & Hagen (1990) | Median duration – 30 (range 1–240) | Rapid onset – 43% Gradual onset – 57% | Severe/excruciating – 100% | Only patients with severe or excruciating pain were classified as having BTP. |
| Fine & Busch (1998) | Mean duration – 52 (range <1–240) | – | Mean intensity – 7/10 (range 3/10–10/10) | |
| Portenoy et al (1999) | – | Median time to peak intensity – 3 min (range 1 sec to 30 min) | Severe/excruciating – 100% | Only patients with severe or excruciating pain were classified as having BTP. |
| Zeppetella et al (2000) | 73% episodes – ≤30 | Rapid onset – 49% Gradual onset – 51% | Slight –16% Moderate – 46% Severe – 36% Excruciating – 2% | |
| Gómez-Batiste et al (2002) | Mean duration – 33.8 (range 1–180) | Rapid onset – 60% Gradual onset – 39% (Not recorded – 1%) | Median intensity – 8/10 (range 2/10–10/10) | |
| Hwang et al (2003) | Median duration – 15 (range 1–120) | Rapid onset – 62% Gradual onset – 38% | Severe/excruciating – 94% | Only patients with severe or excruciating pain were classified as having BTP. |

BTP = breakthrough pain

also signify problems relating to the analgesic regimen (e.g. development of tolerance) (Patt & Ellison 1998).

In spite of the above comments about the diagnosis of breakthrough pain, it has been reported that there is an association between the presence of breakthrough pain and the intensity/frequency of the background pain, i.e. patients with breakthrough pain often have more severe/frequent background pain (Caraceni et al 2004; Portenoy et al, 1999). Indeed, breakthrough pain has been associated with poor overall pain control (Bruera et al 1995, Mercadante et al 1992) and, not surprisingly, with decreased satisfaction with overall pain control (Zeppetella et al 2000).

Some investigators have reported no relationship between clinical features and the different types of breakthrough pain (i.e. spontaneous pain, incident pain, end-of-dose failure) (Portenoy & Hagen 1990). However, others have reported that incident pains tend to be rapid in onset (i.e. incident pain – 76%; spontaneous pain – 52%; end-of-dose failure – 24%), and tend to have a shorter median duration (i.e. incident pain – 20 min; spontaneous pain – 30 min; end-of-dose failure – 30min) (Gómez-Batiste et al 2002).

Similarly, some investigators have reported no relationship between clinical features and the different pathophysiologies of breakthrough pain (i.e. nociceptive, neuropathic) (Portenoy & Hagen 1990). However, others have reported that neuropathic pains tend to have a shorter duration (i.e. neuropathic pain – 91% <30 min; somatic – 69% <30 min; visceral – 62% <30 min) (Zeppetella et al 2000). It should be noted that patients with different pain pathophysiologies tend to report similar pain qualities. Thus, patients with nociceptive pain report 'burning', 'scalding', 'shooting' and 'pricking' pains as much as patients with neuropathic pain (Rasmussen et al 2004).

## 2.4 Other features

### 2.4.1 Chronobiology of breakthrough pain

It appears that there is a circadian variation in the intensity of background pain in patients with cancer (Labrecque & Vanier 1995). Thus various studies have demonstrated a reduction in the intensity of background pain during the night/early morning (Wilder-Smith et al 1992a; Wilder-Smith et al 1992b).

It appears that there is also a circadian variation in the occurrence of breakthrough pain in patients with cancer. For example, Fine & Busch (1998) reported that 86% patients experienced breakthrough pain during the day, whilst only 45% patients experienced breakthrough pain during the night. In addition, various studies have demonstrated a reduction in the usage of breakthrough medication during the night/early morning (Bruera et al 1992, Citron et al 1992).

The reasons for the circadian variation in breakthrough pain have yet to be determined. However, patients are generally less active during the night and so less likely to experience incident pain during this time. Furthermore, there appears to be a circadian variation in the metabolism of certain analgesics (e.g. morphine), which may be of significance with regard to the control of pain (Gourlay et al 1995).

Interestingly, delirium results in an alteration in the circadian variation in breakthrough pain. Thus, Gagnon et al (2001) reported that patients without delirium used breakthrough medication more often during the day, while patients with delirium used breakthrough medication more often during the evening. It should be noted that patients with delirium are often more active during the evening/night and so more likely to experience incident pain at these times.

### 2.4.2 Complications of breakthrough pain

Breakthrough pain can result in a number of physical, psychological and social sequelae:

- **Physical complications** – breakthrough pain may be associated with a variety of physical problems, particularly in patients with volitional (movement-related) incident pain. Such patients have difficulty mobilizing, which may lead them to avoid such movement (see below) (Hwang et al 2003; Portenoy et al 1999). Patients may also have difficulty sleeping, because of the presence of pain (Hwang et al 2003; Portenoy et al 1999)

  As a result of decreased mobility, patients may develop a range of other physical problems, including muscle wasting, joint stiffness, pressure sores, constipation, deep vein thrombosis, and pneumonia. In addition, patients may develop physical problems as a result of the treatment for the breakthrough pain. For example, opioid analgesics are associated with a number of different adverse effects, including somnolence, nausea, vomiting, and dizziness.

- **Psychological complications** – the presence of breakthrough pain has been linked to the presence of 'mood disturbance' (Hwang et al 2003), anxiety (Portenoy et al 1999), and depression (Portenoy et al 1999). The aetiology of these problems include the presence of pain, the "meaning" of the pain, and the physical, and social complications of the pain.

- **Social complications** – breakthrough pain may be associated with a variety of social problems, particularly in patients with volitional (movement-related) incident pain. Such patients may have difficulty undertaking the activities of daily living, which may necessitate increased input from both non-professional and professional carers.

Moreover, patients may be unable to work, which may result in financial hardship for themselves and their dependants. Patients may also have difficulty socializing, because of the presence of pain (Hwang *et al* 2003; Portenoy *et al* 1999).

It can be seen that the presence of breakthrough pain can have a significant negative impact on quality of life (Hwang *et al* 2003; Portenoy *et al*, 1999). The degree of interference seems to be related to the characteristics of the breakthrough pain: patients with spontaneous pain (Portenoy *et al* 1999) or severe pain (Swanwick *et al* 2001) may experience particular problems. In addition, the ability to cope with breakthrough pain seems to be related to the underlying aetiology of the breakthrough pain: patients with cancer-related pain (with all the associated implications) may have more problems coping than patients with cancer treatment-related pain (Foley 1985).

# References

Bruera, E., Macmillan, K., Kuehn, N., Miller, M.J. (1992). Circadian distribution of extra doses of narcotic analgesics in patients with cancer pain: a preliminary report. *Pain*, **49**: 311–314.

Bruera, E., Schoeller, T., Wenk, R., et al. (1995). A prospective multicenter assessment of the Edmonton Staging System for cancer pain. *Journal of Pain and Symptom Management*, **10**: 348–355.

Caraceni, A., Martini, C., Zecca, E., et al. (2004). Breakthrough pain characteristics and syndromes in patients with cancer pain. An international survey. *Palliative Medicine*, **18**: 177–183.

Citron, M.L., Kalra, JM., Seltzer, V.L., Chen, S., et al. (1992). Patient-controlled analgesia for cancer pain: a long term study of inpatient and outpatient use. Cancer *Investigation*, **10**: 335–341.

Davies, A. (2005). Current thinking in cancer breakthrough pain management. *European Journal of Palliative Care*, **12** (Suppl): 4–6.

Fine, P.G., Busch, M.A. (1998). Characterization of breakthrough pain by hospice patients and their caregivers. *Journal of Pain and Symptom Management*, **16**: 179–183.

Foley, K.M. (1985). The treatment of cancer pain. *New England Journal of Medicine*, **313**: 84–95.

Gagnon, B., Lawlor, P.G., Mancini I.L., Pereira, J.L., et al. (2001). The impact of delirium on the circadian distribution of breakthrough analgesia in advanced cancer patients. *Journal of Pain and Symptom Management*, **22**: 826–833.

Gómez-Batiste, X., Madrid, F., Moreno, F., et al. (2002). Breakthrough cancer pain: prevalence and characteristics in patients in Catalonia, Spain. *Journal of Pain and Symptom Management*, **24**: 45–52.

Gourlay, G.K., Plummer, J.L., Cherry, D.A. (1995). Chronopharmacokinetic variability in plasma morphine concentrations following oral doses of morphine solution. *Pain*, **61**: 375–381.

Hwang, S.S., Chang, V.T., Kasimis, B. (2003). Cancer breakthrough pain characteristics and responses to treatment at a VA medical center. *Pain*, **101**: 55–64.

Labrecque, G., Vanier, M.C. (1995). Biological rhythms in pain and in the effects of opioid analgesics. *Pharmacology and Therapeutics*, **68**: 129–147.

Mercadante ,S., Maddaloni, S., Roccella, S., Salvaggio, L. (1992). Predictive factors in advanced cancer pain treated only by analgesics. *Pain*, **50**: 151–155.

Patt, R.B., Ellison, N.M. (1998). Breakthrough pain in cancer patients: characteristics, prevalence, and treatment. *Oncology* (Huntington), **12**: 1035–1052.

Portenoy, R.K., Hagen, N.A. (1990). Breakthrough pain: definition, prevalence and characteristics. *Pain*, **41**: 273–281.

Portenoy, R.K. (1997). Treatment of temporal variations in chronic cancer pain. *Seminars in Oncology*, **5** (SUPPL 16): 7–12.

Portenoy, R.K., Payne, D., Jacobsen, P. (1999). Breakthrough pain: characteristics and impact in patients with cancer pain. *Pain*, **81**: 129–134.

Portenoy, R.K., Forbes, K., Lussier, D., Hanks, G. (2004). Difficult pain problems: an integrated approach. In Doyle, D., Hanks, G., Cherny, N., Calman, K., ed. *Oxford Textbook of Palliative Medicine* (3rd edn), Oxford University Press, Oxford, 438–458.

Rasmussen, P.V., Sindrup, S.H., Jensen, T.S., Bach, F.W. (2004). Symptoms and signs in patients with suspected neuropathic pain. *Pain*, **110**: 461–469.

Simmonds, M.A. (1999). Management of breakthrough pain due to cancer. *Oncology (Huntington)*, **13**: 1103–1108.

Swanwick, M., Haworth, M., Lennard, R.F. (2001). The prevalence of episodic pain in cancer: a survey of hospice patients on admission. *Palliative Medicine*, **15**: 9–18.

Wilder-Smith, C.H., Schimke, J., Bettiga, A. (1992a). Circadian pain responses with tramadol (T), a short-acting opioid and alpha-adrenergic agonist, and morphine (M) in cancer pain: Presented at the 5th International Conference on Chronopharmacology, July 1992.

Wilder-Smith, C.H., Wilder-Smith, O.H. (1992b). Diurnal patterns of pain in cancer patients during treatment with long-acting opioid. Presented at the 5th International Conference on Chronopharmacology, July 1992.

Zeppetella, G., O'Doherty, C.A., Collins, S. (2000). Prevalence and characteristics of breakthrough pain in cancer patients admitted to a hospice. *Journal of Pain and Symptom Management*, **20**: 87–92.

# Chapter 3

# Assessment

Diane Laverty & Andrew Davies

## 3.1 Introduction

Successful management of breakthrough pain depends on adequate assessment, appropriate treatment, and adequate reassessment (i.e. assessment of the treatment) (Davies 2002). Inadequate assessment may lead to ineffective treatment, or even inappropriate treatment. Similarly, inadequate reassessment may lead to the continuance of ineffective/inappropriate treatment (and continuance of pain).

The objectives of assessment are to determine the aetiology of the pain (e.g. cancer-related, non cancer-related), the pathophysiology of the pain (i.e. nociceptive, neuropathic, mixed), and factors that would indicate/contraindicate particular treatment strategies (e.g. performance status, comorbidity). Assessment of breakthrough pain is essentially the same as the assessment of background pain.

## 3.2 Assement procedure

The assessment of pain primarily depends on basic clinical skills, i.e. taking a history and performing an examination (Davies 2002). It is important to take a general history, as well as a pain history. In particular, patients should be screened for psychological, spiritual, and social factors that may be contributing to their experience of pain (the concept of 'total pain') (Twycross 1994). Similarly, it is important to perform a general examination, as well as an examination of the painful area. Investigations can be extremely useful in the assessment of pain. Nevertheless, investigations should only be viewed as a part of the assessment process rather than the main focus of the assessment process. Thus, investigations may produce both false negative results and false positive results.

All patients require a detailed pain history to be taken. The features of the pain that need to be determined include (Foley 2004):

- Onset of pain.
- Temporal pattern of pain – it is important to determine the temporal pattern of the pain, particularly the duration of pain, since it will determine the suitability of certain symptomatic treatments.
- Site of pain.

- Radiation of pain.
- Quality (character) of pain – the quality of the pain may help to determine the aetiology of the pain. However, studies suggest that patients with different pain pathophysiologies tend to report similar pain qualities. Thus, patients with nociceptive pain report 'burning', 'scalding', 'shooting' and 'pricking' pains as much as patients with neuropathic pain. (Rasmussen et al 2004).
- Intensity (severity) of pain – it is important to determine the baseline pain intensity, as this will serve as a marker of the response to treatment (see below).
- Exacerbating factors.
- Relieving factors.
- Response to analgesics – it is essential to determine the response to previous analgesics, particularly to opioid analgesics.
- Response to other interventions – it is essential to determine the response to previous anticancer treatment and non-pharmacological interventions.
- Associated physical symptoms – the presence of other symptoms may help to determine the aetiology of the pain. For example, the presence of neurological symptoms suggests an underlying neuropathic component to the pain (e.g. sensory disturbance) (Bennett 2001).
- Associated psychological symptoms.
- Interference with activities of daily living – it is important to ascertain the global impact of the pain. (Activities of daily living can be used as a surrogate marker of the response to treatment).

All patients require a thorough examination to be performed. The examinations should include a neurological examination of the relevant area, since the presence of neurological signs suggests an underlying neuropathic component to the pain (Bennett 2001). It can be useful to reproduce the patient's pain by using so-called 'provocative manoeuvres' (e.g. palpation, passive movement) (Hagen 1999). However, it is important that the benefits of such manoeuvres (i.e. improved understanding of the pain) outweigh the 'costs' of these manoeuvres (i.e. causation of pain).

It should be noted that many patients have more than one type of breakthrough pain (Portenoy & Hagen 1990; Portenoy et al 1999). Each breakthrough pain should be individually assessed, since each breakthrough pain may require a different form of treatment.

## 3.3 Reassessment procedure

The primary objective of reassessment is to determine the efficacy and tolerability of any therapeutic intervention. A further objective of reassessment is the identification of significant changes in the breakthrough pain. For example, increasing pain in a bone may represent impending fracture of that bone (which may necessitate a more intensive therapeutic intervention e.g. surgical stabilization).

Various outcome measures have been used to assess the efficacy of therapeutic interventions, including: a) intensity of pain; b) distress of pain; c) pain relief; d) satisfaction with treatment; e) improvement in function; and f) improvement in quality of life (Davies 2002). The different outcome measures relate to diffferent aspects of the pain. Consequently there is often a poor correlation between the results obtained with different outcome measures. For example, in one study involving oncology patients, the percentage of subjects that were 'inadequately treated' varied from 16–91% depending on the specific outcome measure used (de Wit et al 1999).

All of the aforementioned outcome measures have limitations. For example, pain relief is related to the change in pain intensity over a period of time, i.e. it is dependent on the patient's recollection of the baseline pain intensity. There is little consensus on the specific outcome measure that should be used to assess treatment response (de Wit et al 1999). Nevertheless, it is important that a suitable outcome measure is used to assess treatment response in all patients (Davies 2002).

Outcome measures are usually based on a verbal rating scale, a numerical rating scale, or a visual analogue scale (Figure 3.1). Studies have shown a good correlation between the results obtained with these different scales (McQuay & Moore 1998): the relationship between the results obtained with these different scales is shown in Table 3.1. However, patients with advanced cancer often have difficulty in completing such outcome measures. For example, in one study involving palliative care inpatients, 45% of the subjects were unable to complete any of the outcome measures (mainly because of cognitive impairment) (Shannon et al 1995).

It should be noted that studies suggest that the formal measurement of pain leads to the improved management of pain. For example, in one study involving oncology out-patients, subjects whose outcome measures were reviewed were more likely to have had an improvement in their background pain intensity at follow up than subjects whose outcome measures were unavailable for review (Trowbridge et al 1997).

## 3.4 Assessment tools

A number of different tools have been developed for the assessment of cancer-related pain (Caraceni et al 2002). However, these tools invariably focus on the background pain rather than the breakthrough pain. Moreover, most of these tools provide little, or no, information about the breakthrough pain.

## Fig 3.1 Examples of pain measurement scales

- Verbal rating scale, e.g. McGill Pain Questionnaire (Melzack, 1975).

  **No pain; mild; discomforting; distressing; horrible; excruciating**

- Numerical rating scale, e.g. Brief Pain Inventory (Daut et al, 1983).

  A. Pain intensity

  **0   1   2   3   4   5   6   7   8   9   10**

  No                                    Pain as bad
  pain                                  as you can
                                        imagine

  B. Pain relief

  **0% 10% 20% 30% 40% 50% 60% 70% 80% 90% 100%**

  No                                    Complete
  relief                                relief

- Visual analogue scale, e.g. Memorial Pain Assessment Card
  (Fishman et al 1987).

  A. Pain intensity

  **LEAST** ——————————————— **WORST**
  possible                          possible
  pain                              pain

  B. Pain relief

  **NO** ——————————————— **COMPLETE**
  relief                            relief
  of pain                           of pain

## Table 3.1 Correlation between results of different pain measurement scales

| Verbal rating scale | Numerical rating scale (0–10) (Serlin et al 1995) | Visual analogue scale (100 mm) (Collins et al 1997) |
| --- | --- | --- |
| None | 0 | – |
| Mild | 1–4 | – |
| Moderate | 5–6 | >30 mm (mean 49) |
| Severe | 7–10 | >54 mm (mean 75) |

## Fig 3.2 Breakthrough pain assessment algorithm (courtesy of Russell Portenoy)

**Breakthrough pain assessment algorithm**

**A. Determining the presence of persistent baseline pain**

1. Does your pain currently have a component you would describe as 'constant' or 'almost constant', or would it be constant or almost constant if not for the treatment you are receiving?

   If **Yes**, go to question 2 (patients taking an opioid regimen for >12 h/day), or question 3 (patients taking an opioid regimen for <12 h/day).

   *If No, stop. Patient does not have persistent baseline pain.*

2. **For patients taking an opioid regimen for >12 h/day**

   a) Have you had any pain during the past week?

      If **Yes**, go to question 2b.

      If **No**, patient has controlled baseline pain. Continue to section B

   b) How would you judge your baseline pain, on average during the past week?

              Mild  Moderate  Severe  Excruciating

      If **mild** or **moderate**, patient has controlled baseline pain. Continue to section B.

      *If severe or excruciating, stop. Patient has uncontrolled baseline pain.*

3. **For patients taking an opioid regimen for <12 h/day**

   a) Have you had any pain during the past week?

      If **Yes**, go to question 3b.

      *If No, stop. Patient does not have baseline pain.*

   b) Did you feel this pain for more than half the time that you were awake?

      If **Yes,** continue to question 3c.

      *If No, stop. Patient has transient pains.*

   c) How would you judge your baseline pain, on average during the past week?

              Mild  Moderate  Severe  Excruciating

      If **mild** or **moderate**, patient has controlled baseline pain. Continue to section B.

      *If severe or excruciating, stop. Patient has uncontrolled baseline pain.*

**B. Assessing the nature of the baseline pain**

Further questions about the baseline pain.

**C. Determining the presence of breakthrough pain**

1. Do you also experience temporary flares of severe or excruciating pain?

   If **Yes**, patient has breakthrough pain. Continue with the remainder of this questionnaire to characterize the breakthrough pain.

   *If No, stop. Patient has controlled baseline pain without breakthrough pain.*

**D. Assessing the nature of the breakthrough pain**

Further questions about the breakthrough pain (see text).

**Fig 3.3 Episodic pain documentation sheet (reproduced with permission from Zeppetella & Ribeiro [2002]).**

Patient name:_____ Date:_____

Each pain should be marked on a separate sheet

**Location**

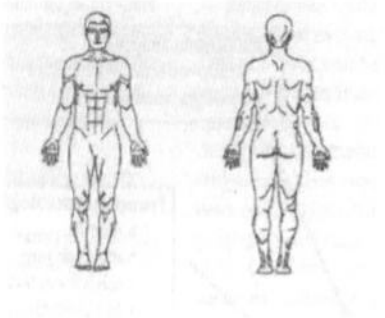

**Severity**

| | |
|---|---|
| Mild | [ ] |
| Moderate | [ ] |
| Severe | [ ] |
| Excruciating | [ ] |

**Type**

| | |
|---|---|
| A. No background pain | [ ] |
| B. Controlled background pain | [ ] |
| C. Uncontrolled background pain | [ ] |

| | |
|---|---|
| 0. No scheduled analgesia | [ ] |
| 1. Insufficient scheduled analgesia | [ ] |
| 2. Sufficient scheduled analgesia | [ ] |

**Temporal characteristics**
Daily frequency: _____

Weekly frequency (if less than daily) _____

Onset:      Gradual [ ]   Sudden [ ]

Time course
   Time to max intensity (minutes) _____     Total duration (minutes) _____

**Precipitating event**

| | |
|---|---|
| None (spontaneous) | [ ] |
| Incident | [ ] |
| Non-volitional | [ ] |

**Pathophysiology**

| | |
|---|---|
| Somatic | [ ] |
| Visceral | [ ] |
| Neuropathic | [ ] |
| Mixed | [ ] |
| Unknown | [ ] |

**Predictable**

| | |
|---|---|
| Yes | [ ] |
| No | [ ] |

**Aetiology**

| | |
|---|---|
| Disease related | [ ] |
| Treatment related | [ ] |
| Unrelated to disease/treatment | [ ] |

**Notes**

Portenoy and Hagen developed the Breakthrough Pain Questionnaire to specifically assess breakthrough pain (Portenoy & Hagen 1990). It has been used in a number of clinical studies (Portenoy & Hagen 1990; Portenoy et al 1999), although it does not appear to have been formally validated (Patt & Ellison 1998). In addition, the Breakthrough Pain Questionnaire has evolved over the intervening years (Russell Portenoy, personal communication).

The Breakthrough Pain Questionnaire enables the healthcare professional to identify patients with breakthrough pain, as well as to collect information about the nature of the breakthrough pain and of the background pain. The criteria for diagnosing breakthrough pain are: 1) presence of background pain, i.e. patient has pain that has

Figure 3.3 reproduced with permission from Zeppetella, G., Ribeiro, M.D.C (2002). Episodic pain in patients with advanced cancer. *American Journal of Hospice and Palliative Care*, **19**(4): 267–276.

been there for more than half the waking time during the previous week, or the patient has been taking regular opioid analgesics for more than half of the days during the previous week; 2) presence of controlled background pain, i.e. patient has pain that has been rated as 'absent', 'mild' or 'moderate' (but not 'severe') for more than half of the time; and 3) occurrence of one or more 'severe or excruciating episodes of pain' during the previous day (Portenoy et al 1999). A suitable breakthrough pain assessment algorithm is shown in Figure 3.2.

It should be noted that patients with no background pain but who have severe or excruciating episodes of pain are classified as having 'transitory pains' (Portenoy et al 1999). Similarly, patients that have poorly controlled background pain, and severe or excruciating episodes of pain are simply classified as having 'uncontrolled pain' (Portenoy et al 1999).

Other investigators have also developed tools specifically to assess breakthrough pain. For example, Zeppetella has produced an episodic (breakthrough) pain documentation sheet for use within his palliative care unit (Figure 3.3) (Zeppetella & Ribeiro 2002).

# References

Bennett, M. (2001). The LANSS Pain Scale: the Leeds assessment of neuropathic symptoms and signs. *Pain*, **92**: 147–157.

Caraceni, A., Cherny, N., Fainsinger, R., et al. (2002). Pain measurement tools and methods in clinical research in palliative care: recommendations of an Expert Working Group of the European Association of Palliative Care. *Journal of Pain and Symptom Management*, **23**: 239–255.

Collins, S.L., Moore, A., McQuay, H.J. (1997). The visual analogue pain intensity scale: what is moderate pain in millimetres? *Pain*, **72**: 95–97.

Daut, R.L., Cleeland, C.S., Flanery, R.C. (1983). Development of the Wisconsin Brief Pain Questionnaire to assess pain in cancer and other diseases. *Pain*, **17**: 197–210.

Davies, A. (2002). The assessment and measurement of physical pain. In Hillier, R., Finlay, I., Miles, A., ed. *The Effective Management of Cancer Pain* (2nd edn). Aesculapius Medical Press, London, 23–28.

de Wit, R., van Dam, F., Abu-Saad, H.H., et al. (1999). Empirical comparison of commonly used measures to evaluate pain treatment in cancer patients with chronic pain. *Journal of Clinical Oncology*, **17**: 1280–1287.

Fishman, B., Pasternak, S., Wallenstein, S.L., et al. (1987). The Memorial Pain Assessment Card: a valid instrument for the evaluation of cancer pain. *Cancer*, **60**: 1151–1158.

Foley, K.M. (2004). Acute and chronic cancer pain syndromes. In Doyle, D., Hanks G., Cherny, N., Calman, K., ed. *Oxford Textbook of Palliative Medicine* (3rd edn). Oxford University Press, Oxford, 298–316.

Hagen, N.A. (1999). Reproducing a cancer patient's pain on physical examination: bedside provocative maneuvers. *Journal of Pain and Symptom Management*, **18**: 406–411.

McQuay, H.J., Moore, R.A. (1998). *An Evidence-based Resource for Pain Relief.* Oxford University Press, Oxford.

Melzack, R. (1975). The McGill Pain Questionnaire: major properties and scoring methods. *Pain,* **1**: 277–299.

Patt R.B., Ellison, N.M. (1998). Breakthrough pain in cancer patients: characteristics, prevalence, and treatment. *Oncology (Huntington),* **12**: 1035–1052.

Portenoy, R.K., Hagen, N.A. (1990). Breakthrough pain: definition, prevalence and characteristics. *Pain,* **41**: 273–281.

Portenoy, R.K., Payne, D., Jacobsen, P. (1999). Breakthrough pain: characteristics and impact in patients with cancer pain. *Pain,* **81**: 129–134.

Rasmussen, P.V., Sindrup, S.H., Jensen, T.S., Bach, F.W. (2004). Symptoms and signs in patients with suspected neuropathic pain. *Pain,* **110**: 461–469.

Serlin, R.C., Mendoza, T.R., Nakamura, Y., et al. (1995). When is cancer pain mild, moderate or severe? Grading pain severity by its interference with function. *Pain,* **61**: 277–284.

Shannon, M.M., Ryan, M.A., D'Agostino, N., Brescia, F.J. (1995). Assessment of pain in advanced cancer patients. *Journal of Pain and Symptom Management,* **10**: 274–278.

Trowbridge, R., Dugan, W., Jay, S.J., et al. (1997). Determining the effectiveness of a clinical practice intervention in improving the control of pain in outpatients with cancer. *Academic Medicine,* **72**: 798–800.

Twycross, R. (1994). *Pain Relief in Advanced Cancer.* Churchill Livingstone, Edinburgh.

Zeppetella, G., Ribeiro, M.D. (2002). Episodic pain in patients with advanced cancer. *American Journal of Hospice and Palliative Care,* **19**: 267–276.

# Chapter 4

# General principles of management

Andrew Davies

## 4.1 Introduction

Breakthrough pain is not a single entity, but a spectrum of very different entities. The treatment of breakthrough pain depends on a variety of pain-related factors, including the aetiology of the pain, the pathophysiology of the pain, and the characteristics of the pain. Moreover, it depends on a variety of patient-related factors, including the stage of the disease and the performance status of the patient (Mercadante & Arcuri 1998). Thus, treatment is highly individualized (Patt & Ellison 1998).

The management of breakthrough pain involves: a) assessment; b) treatment of the cause of the pain; c) treatment of the pain *per se* (symptomatic treatment); and d) reassessment. Chapter 3 describes the assessment of breakthrough pain in more detail. This chapter will discuss the general principles of the treatment of breakthrough pain. Subsequent chapters describe the symptomatic treatment of breakthrough pain in more detail.

## 4.2 Management strategies

The optimal treatment for all types of breakthrough pain is management of the underlying disease and/or the underlying pathological process. It should be noted, however, that although these types of intervention have been shown to be very effective in managing background pain, they have generally not been evaluated for their effectiveness in managing breakthrough pain (e.g. radiotheraphy, bisphosphonates) (Mercadante et al 2002). Nevertheless, there is anecdotal evidence that some of these interventions may also be effective in managing some instances of breakthrough pain (Mercadante et al 2001).

The symptomatic management of breakthrough pain includes:

- Pharmacological treatment of pain:
  1. Modification of the background analgesic regimen.
     a) Increase dose of analgesic drugs.
     b) Addition of analgesic drugs.
     c) Addition of co-analgesic drugs.

**Table 4.1** Relieving factors of breakthrough pain in studies applying recognized criteria for breakthrough pain

| Study | Relieving factors | | | Comments |
|---|---|---|---|---|
| | Medication | Other strategies | No relieving factors | |
| Portenoy & Hagen (1990) | 44% | 44% | 12% | Some patients had more than one relieving factor. |
| Portenoy et al (1999) | 61% | 26% | 13% | |
| Hwang et al (2003) | 54% | 26% | 20% | Data refer to initial assessment (see text). |

2. Use of breakthrough ('rescue') analgesics.
   a) Non-opioid analgesics.
   b) Opioid analgesics.
   c) Other agents, e.g. nitrous oxide, midazolam.
 • Non-pharmacological treatment of pain.

A variety of non-pharmacological methods may be useful in treating breakthrough pain, e.g. rubbing/massage (Fine & Busch 1998; Swanwick et al 2001), application of heat (Fine & Busch 1998; Swanwick et al 2001), application of cold (Fine & Busch 1998; Petzke et al 1999), transcutaneous nerve stimulation (TENS) (Zeppetella & Ribeiro 2003), distraction techniques (Portenoy 1997; Petzke et al 1999), and relaxation techniques (Portenoy 1997; Fine & Busch 1998).

Table 4.1 shows the relieving factors reported by patients in studies applying standard criteria for the diagnosis of breakthrough pain (Portenoy & Hagen 1990; Portenoy et al 1999; Hwang et al 2003). It can be seen that only 44–61% of patients reported that their medication relieved breakthrough pain. Nevertheless, Hwang et al have shown that alterations in medication can lead to improvements in breakthrough pain (Hwang et al 2003). Thus, 54% of patients reported that their medication relieved breakthrough pain at baseline, whilst 83% of patients reported that their medication relieved breakthrough pain after 1 week of intervention. It should be noted that patients often report more than one relieving factor, e.g. a non-pharmacological intervention and a pharmacological intervention (Portenoy & Hagen 1990; Swanwick et al 2001).

## 4.3 **Management of spontaneous pain**

The symptomatic management of spontaneous pain involves modification of the background analgesic regimen, and use of breakthrough medication. The options for modification of the background analgesia are:

- Increase the dose of the analgesic – this strategy can be effective in reducing the frequency and/or severity of breakthrough pain (Portenoy 1997). It has been suggested that the dose is initially increased by 25–50% (Portenoy 1997). However, this strategy is often limited by the development of side effects. Nevertheless, some authorities have suggested that all patients should be given a therapeutic trial of this strategy (Portenoy, 1997).

One of the major restrictions to increasing the dose of opioid analgesics is the development of opioid-related drowsiness. Bruera et al have reported that this problem can be relieved by the concurrent use of methylphenidate (a psychostimulant) (Bruera et al 1992). An alternative strategy would be opioid substitution/opioid switching (also known as opioid rotation) (Cherny et al 2001). It should be noted that opioid substitution/opioid switching may also be useful in managing other opioid-related side effects (Cherny et al 2001).

- Addition of analgesic drugs – the rationale for this strategy is that the addition of another analgesic drug may result in a better effect/side-effect profile than increasing the dose of the original analgesic drug.
- Addition of co-analgesic drugs – this strategy can be effective in reducing the frequency and/or severity of specific types of breakthrough pain. For example, neuropathic pain may be eased in many cases by the use of certain groups of drugs (e.g. anticonvulsant drugs, antidepressant drugs) (Portenoy et al 2004).

Nevertheless, in many cases, treatment of spontaneous pain relies on the use of breakthrough medication, e.g. fast-acting, short-lasting opioid analgesics (see below).

## 4.4 Management of incident pain

The management of incident pain includes treatment of precipitants of the pain, as well as symptomatic treatment of the pain. The precipitants of incident pain are extremely varied (Table 1.2), and only some of these precipitants may be amenable to specific treatment (e.g. opioids to suppress coughing) (Portenoy 1997).

Movement-related (volitional incident) pain, secondary to metastatic bone disease, is a common phenomenon. Moreover, studies suggest that this can be the most difficult type of breakthrough pain to manage (Hwang et al 2003). In some cases, it may be possible to perform surgical stabilization of the relevant bone(s) (see Figure 4.1a/b) (Mercadante et al 2002). Alternatively, it may be possible to use an orthotic device to stabilize the relevant bone(s) (see Figure 4.2) (Mercadante & Arcuri 1998). However, many patients will benefit from strategies to minimize the amount of movement required, such as provision of simple adaptations to their surroundings and provision of additional practical support with the activities of daily living (Mercadante & Arcuri 1998).

The symptomatic management of incident pain involves modification of the background analgesic regimen and use of breakthrough medication. The options for modification of the background analgesia are:

- Increase the dose of the analgesic – (see Management of spontaneous pain). Mercadante et al (2004b) reported that increasing the dose of regular opioid was effective in managing movement-related (volitional incident) pain in a group of patients with bone metastases. Moreover, they reported that increasing the dose of regular opioid was generally well tolerated by this group of patients.

- Addition of analgesic drugs – (see Management of spontaneous pain).

- Addition of co-analgesic drugs – (see Management of spontaneous pain). For example, pain on defaecation may be eased in some cases by the use of softening laxatives, or in other cases by the use of antispasmodic drugs. Similarly, pain on swallowing may be eased in some cases by the use of coating agents, or in other cases by the use of local anaesthetics.

Nevertheless, in many cases, treatment of incident pain relies on the use of breakthrough medication. In some cases, the pain is predictable, and so it is possible to take the breakthrough medication in advance.

### Fig 4.1 X-rays demonstrating surgical stabilization of a lytic bone metastasis

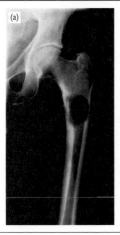
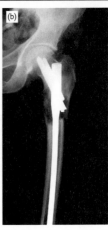

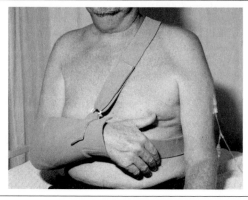

**Fig 4.2 Orthotic device (Polysling®) for supporting/ immobilizing the upper arm**

However, it is important that the breakthrough medication is taken far enough in advance of the relevant activity. For example, the time to onset of effect for oral morphine is 20–30 min (Twycross et al 1998) and the time to maximum effect is 60 min (Mercadante et al 2002). Thus, oral morphine should be given at least 30 min, and probably 60 min, before the relevant activity.

## 4.5 Management of end-of-dose failure

The management of end-of-dose failure involves modification of the background analgesic regimen (Mercadante et al 2002). The options are:

- Increase the dose of the analgesic – this is the recommended strategy for treating end-of-dose failure with most opioid analgesics (e.g. morphine, oxycodone) (Hanks et al 2001). This strategy is invariably effective, although the increase in dosage may lead to an increase in side effects. Indeed, some patients may be unable to tolerate an increase in dosage (Simmonds 1999).

- Increase the frequency of the analgesic – this is a recommended strategy for treating end-of-dose failure with transdermal fentanyl (see below) (Breitbart et al 2000). This strategy has been used for treating end-of-dose failure with other opioids, although it is generally not recommended (Hanks et al 2001).

In most patients, the duration of action of transdermal fentanyl is 72 hr. Nevertheless, in some (3–43%) patients, the duration of action of transdermal fentanyl is somewhere between 48 and 72 hr (Payne et al 1995; Grond et al 1997). It has been recommended that patients who are pain controlled for 48 hr, but require breakthrough medication between 48 and 72 hr, should replace their patch every 48 hr rather than every 72 hr (rather than increasing the dose of the patch) (Breitbart et al 2000).

• Provision of additional analgesic drugs/other pain-relief methods – in some cases, the aforementioned strategies are either not possible or lead to intolerable side effects. In such cases, the provision of additional analgesic drugs and/or other pain-relief methods are required to control the background pain.

## 4.6 Breakthrough ('rescue'/'supplemental') medication

In theory, any fast-acting analgesic can be used to treat breakthrough pain (i.e. non-opioid analgesics, opioid analgesics, adjuvant analgesics) (Mercadante & Arcuri 1998). Nevertheless, opioid preparations are the mainstay of the pharmacological management of breakthrough pain. However, opioid preparations will only be effective if the breakthrough pain is an opioid responsive pain. Moreover, individual opioid preparations will only be effective if the pharmacokinetic profile of the preparation mirrors the temporal pattern of the pain. It should be noted that response (efficacy, tolerability) to individual opioid preparations varies from person to person, and may vary over time within the same person.

The World Health Organization (WHO) guidelines promote the use of the oral route for the management of cancer pain (WHO 1996). However, although the oral route is usually effective for background pain, it is generally less effective for the management of breakthrough pain. The oral route is associated with a delayed onset of action (~20–30 min for oral morphine) (Twycross et al 1998) and a delayed peak effect (~ 60 min for oral morphine) (Mercadante et al 2002). In an attempt to overcome this issue a variety of alternative routes have been utilized including the oral transmucosal (Gardner-Nix 2001), intravenous (Mercadante et al 2004a), subcutaneous (Enting et al 2005), intranasal (Pavis et al 2002), and intrapulmonary routes (Zeppetella 2000a). Unfortunately, although these routes are usually very effective, the generic use of these routes is limited by practical issues including the availability of trained personnel, suitable drug preparations, and suitable drug delivery systems. Subsequent chapters describe these routes of administration in more detail.

In the past, it has been recommended that the opioid used to treat breakthrough pain should generally be the same as the opioid used to treat background pain (Patt & Ellison 1998). However, there are no compelling reasons for using the same opioid, and the decision to use an opioid should be based on its pharmacokinetic profile rather than its pharmacodynamic profile. Traditionally, it was also recommended that the dose of opioid to treat breakthrough pain should be a fixed ratio of the daily dose of opioid to treat the background pain (Patt & Ellison 1998). However, the ratio varied significantly between guidelines (e.g. 1/24 to 1/6 daily dose) (Cleary 1997). Data from recent studies suggest that there is no relationship between the dose required to control breakthrough pain and the dose required to control background pain (Coluzzi et al 2001). Thus, the dose of breakthrough medication should be titrated in the same manner as the dose of background medication (Mercadante et al 2002).

The side effects associated with taking a breakthrough dose of opioid are similar to those associated with taking any dose of opioid, e.g. somnolence, nausea, vomiting, and dizziness (Coluzzi et al 2001). In the United Kingdom, guidelines on driving and opioid medication state that in view of the risk of somnolence 'you must not drive on days where you have had to take extra (breakthrough or rescue) doses of a strong painkiller' (Pease et al 2004).

## 4.7 Other issues

### 4.7.1 Prescription of breakthrough medication

Studies suggest that patients are frequently not prescribed breakthrough medication. For example, Ferrell et al (1999) reported that 27% of patients in their study had not been prescribed breakthrough medication. Other authors have reported even higher levels of non-prescription (i.e. 38–57%) (Weber & Huber 1999; Zeppetella et al 2000b; Lawrie et al 2003). Ferrell et al (1999) also found that patients that had been prescribed breakthrough medication in their study had had inappropriate limitations imposed on the frequency of use of the breakthrough medication. Thus, only 29% patients were told that they could use the breakthrough medication the recommended 1–2 hrly (if required).

### 4.7.2 Concordance with breakthrough medication

Non-concordance (also known as non-compliance) with prescribed medication appears to be common amongst patients with cancer. For example, Zeppetella et al (1999) reported that 44% of homecare patients were not taking their medication, particularly their analgesics (i.e. non-opioids, opioids), as prescribed.

Similarly, Ferrell et al (1999) reported that only 3% of patients were taking their breakthrough medication as prescribed. Specifically, 96% of patients were taking too low a dose, 3% of patients were taking the prescribed dose, and 1% of patients were taking too high a dose. Indeed, the mean dose taken was only 21% of the dose prescribed. The reasons for the non-concordance in this study were unclear although other studies have cited lack of effect, adverse events, concerns about adverse events, difficulty in taking the medication, and lack of knowledge about the medication (Zeppetella 1999).

**Table 4.2 Acceptability of different routes of administration of breakthrough medication for mild-to-moderate pain (Walker et al 2003)**

| Route | Acceptability of route for mild to moderate pain | | | Reasons for unacceptability |
|---|---|---|---|---|
| | Yes (%) | Possibly (%) | No (%) | |
| Oral | 97 | 1 | 2 | Slow onset of action |
| Rectal | 24 | 19 | 57 | Dignity, previous bad experience, localized pain/disease, difficult to administer, unpleasant/uncomfortable, 'inappropriate for level of pain' |
| Nasal | 50 | 18 | 32 | Localized pain/disease, difficult to administer, catches back of throat, fear of bad taste/nausea, unpleasant/uncomfortable, unfamiliar/dislike idea |
| Sublingual | 63 | 19 | 18 | Previous bad experience, fear of bad taste/nausea, unfamiliar/dislike idea |
| Transmucosal | 44 | 21 | 35 | Fear of bad taste/nausea, 'childlike', unfamiliar/dislike idea, risk of children taking drug |
| Inhaled | 60 | 19 | 21 | Previous bad experience, localized pain/disease, difficult to administer, fear of bad taste/nausea, unfamiliar/dislike idea |
| Subcutaneous | 52 | 20 | 28 | 'Inappropriate for level of pain', dislike of injections |
| Intramuscular | 33 | 22 | 45 | 'Inappropriate for level of pain', dislike of injections |
| Intravenous | 38 | 23 | 39 | Previous bad experience, 'inappropriate for level of pain', dislike of injections |

Table 4.3 Acceptability of different routes of administration of breakthrough medication for severe pain (Walker et al 2003)

| Route | Acceptability of route for severe pain | | | Reasons for unacceptability |
|---|---|---|---|---|
| | Yes (%) | Possibly (%) | No (%) | |
| Oral | 88 | 4 | 8 | Slow onset of action |
| Rectal | 48 | 10 | 42 | Slow onset of action, dignity, previous bad experience, localized pain/disease, difficult to administer, unpleasant/uncomfortable |
| Nasal | 68 | 14 | 18 | Localized pain/disease, difficult to administer, catches back of throat, fear of bad taste/nausea, unfamiliar/dislike idea |
| Sublingual | 75 | 11 | 14 | Slow onset of action, previous bad experience, fear of bad taste/nausea, unfamiliar/dislike idea |
| Transmucosal | 63 | 12 | 25 | Localized pain/disease, fear of bad taste/nausea, 'childlike', unfamiliar/dislike idea |
| Inhaled | 75 | 9 | 16 | Previous bad experience, localized pain/disease, difficult to administer, fear of bad taste/nausea, unfamiliar/dislike idea |
| Subcutaneous | 87 | 8 | 5 | Dislike of injections |
| Intramuscular | 76 | 12 | 12 | Dislike of injections |
| Intravenous | 83 | 8 | 9 | Previous bad experience, dislike of injections |

Other authors have reported that the use of breakthrough medication depends on the type of breakthrough pain (Gómez-Batiste et al 2002). Patients with incident pain were less likely to use breakthrough medication than those with spontaneous pain or end-of-dose failure. The most likely reason for this phenomenon is that incident pain tends to be of shorter duration than spontaneous pain or end-of-dose failure, and so is less likely to respond to breakthrough medication.

### 4.7.3 Acceptability of breakthrough medication

One factor that may affect concordance is the acceptability of the breakthrough medication. Table 4.2 shows the acceptability of different routes of administration to palliative care patients if the pain was rated as 'mild to moderate' (Walker et al 2003). Similarly, Table 4.3 shows the acceptability of these routes of administration to palliative care patients if the pain was rated as 'severe'. (It should be noted that patients were informed that the onset of pain relief was 5 min for the intravenous route; 10 min for the nasal, sublingual, transmucosal, inhaled, subantaneous and intramuscular routes; and 30 min for the oral and rectal routes.) It can be seen that the acceptability of a route is somewhat dependent on the severity of the pain, i.e. the more severe the pain the more likely the patient will accept an invasive route of administration (Walker et al 2003).

## References

Breitbart, W., Chandler, S., Eagel, B., et al. (2000). An alternative algorithm for dosing transdermal fentanyl for cancer-related pain. *Oncology (Huntington)*, **14**: 695–705.

Bruera, E., Fainsinger, R., MacEachern, T., Hanson, J. (1992). The use of methylphenidate in patients with incident cancer pain receiving regular opiates. A preliminary report. *Pain*, **50**: 75–77.

Cherny, N., Ripamonti, C., Pereira, J. et al. (2001). Strategies to manage the adverse effects of oral morphine: an evidence-based report. *Journal of Clinical Oncology*, **19**: 2542–2554.

Cleary, J.F. (1997). Pharmacokinetic and pharmacodynamic issues in the treatment of breakthrough pain. *Seminars in Oncology*, **24**: (Suppl 16): S16–13–9.

Coluzzi, P.H., Schwartzberg, L., Conroy, Jr J.D., et al. (2001). Breakthrough cancer pain: a randomized trial comparing oral transmucosal fentanyl citrate (OTFC) and morphine sulfate immediate release (MSIR). *Pain*, **91**: 123–130.

Enting, R.H., Mucchiano, C., Oldenmenger, W.H., et al. (2005). The 'Pain Pen' for breakthrough cancer pain: a promising treatment. *Journal of Pain and Symptom Management*, **29**: 213–217.

Ferrell, B.R., Juarez, G., Borneman, T. (1999). Use of routine and breakthrough analgesia in home care. *Oncology Nursing Forum*, **26**: 1655–1661.

Fine, P.G., Busch, M.A. (1998). Characterization of breakthrough pain by hospice patients and their caregivers. *Journal of Pain and Symptom Management*, **16**: 179–183.

Gardner-Nix, J. (2001). Oral transmucosal fentanyl and sufentanil for incident pain. *Journal of Pain and Symptom Management*, **22**: 627–630.

Gómez-Batiste, X., Madrid, F., Moreno, F., et al. (2002). Breakthrough cancer pain: prevalence and characteristics in patients in Catalonia, Spain. *Journal of Pain and Symptom Management*, **24**: 45–52.

Grond, S., Zech, D., Lehmann, K.A., et al. (1997). Transdermal fentanyl in the long-term treatment of cancer pain: a prospective study of 50 patients with advanced cancer of the gastrointestinal tract or the head and neck region. *Pain*, **69**: 191–198.

Hanks, G.W., de Conno, F., Cherny, N., et al. (2001). Morphine and alternative opioids in cancer pain: the EAPC recommendations. *British Journal of Cancer*, **84**: 587–593.

Hwang, S.S., Chang, V.T., Kasimis, B. (2003). Cancer breakthrough pain characteristics and responses to treatment at a VA medical center. *Pain*, **101**: 55–64.

Lawrie, I., Lloyd-Williams, M., Waterhouse, E. (2003). Breakthrough strong opioid analgesia prescription in patients using transdermal fentanyl admitted to a hospice. *American Journal of Hospice and Palliative Care*, **20**: 229–230.

Mercadante, S., Arcuri, E. (1998). Breakthrough pain in cancer patients: pathophysiology and treatment. *Cancer Treatment Reviews*, **24**: 425–432.

Mercadante, S., Villari, P., Ferrera, P., Dabbene, M. (2001). Pamidronate in incident pain due to bone metastases. *Journal of Pain and Symptom Management*, **22**: 630–631.

Mercadante, S., Radbruch, L., Caraceni, A., et al. (2002). Episodic (breakthrough) pain. Consensus Conference of an Expert Working Group of the European Association for Palliative Care. *Cancer*, **94**: 832–839.

Mercadante, S., Villari, P., Ferrera, P. et al. (2004a). Safety and effectiveness of intravenous morphine for episodic (breakthrough) pain using a fixed ratio with the oral daily morphine dose. *Journal of Pain and Symptom Management*, **27**: 352–359.

Mercadante, S., Villari, P., Ferrera, P., Casuccio, A. (2004b). Optimization of opioid therapy for preventing incident pain associated with bone metastases. *Journal of Pain and Symptom Management*, **28**: 505–510.

Patt, R.B., Ellison, N.M. (1998). Breakthrough pain in cancer patients: characteristics, prevalence, and treatment. *Oncology (Huntington)*, **12**: 1035–1052.

Pavis, H., Wilcock, A., Edgecombe, J. et al. (2002). Pilot study of nasal morphine-chitosan for the relief of breakthrough pain in patients with cancer. *Journal of Pain and Symptom Management*, **24**: 598–602.

Payne, R., Chandler, S., Einhaus, M. (1995). Guidelines for the clinical use of transdermal fentanyl. *Anti-Cancer Drugs*, **6**(Suppl 3): 50–53.

41

Pease, N., Taylor, H., Major, H. (2004). Driving advice for palliative care patients taking strong opioid medication. *Palliative Medicine*, **18**: 663–665.

Petzke, F., Radbruch, L., Zech, D., et al. (1999). Temporal presentation of chronic cancer pain: transitory pains on admission to a multidisciplinary pain clinic. *Journal of Pain and Symptom Management*, **17**: 391–401.

Portenoy, R.K., Hagen, N.A. (1990). Breakthrough pain: definition, prevalence and characteristics. *Pain*, **41**: 273–281.

Portenoy, R.K. (1997). Treatment of temporal variations in chronic cancer pain. *Seminars in Oncology*, **5** (Suppl 16): 7–12.

Portenoy, R.K., Payne, D., Jacobsen, P. (1999). Breakthrough pain: characteristics and impact in patients with cancer pain. *Pain*, **81**: 129–134.

Portenoy, R.K., Forbes, K., Lussier, D., Hanks, G. (2004). Difficult pain problems: an integrated approach. In Doyle D, Hanks G, Cherny N, Calman K, ed. *Oxford Textbook of Palliative Medicine* (3rd edn), Oxford University Press, Oxford, 438–458.

Simmonds, M.A. (1999). Management of breakthrough pain due to cancer. *Oncology (Huntington)*, **13**: 1103–1108.

Swanwick, M., Haworth, M., Lennard, R.F. (2001). The prevalence of episodic pain in cancer: a survey of hospice patients on admission. *Palliative Medicine*, **15**: 9–18.

Twycross, R., Wilcock, A., Thorp, S. (1998). *Palliative Care Formulary*. Radcliffe Medical Press Ltd, Abingdon.

Walker, G., Wilcock, A., Manderson, C., et al. (2003). The acceptability of different routes of administration of analgesia for breakthrough pain. *Palliative Medicine*, **17**: 219–221.

Weber, M., Huber, C. (1999). Documentation of severe pain, opioid doses, and opioid-related side effects in outpatients with cancer: a retrospective study. *Journal of Pain and Symptom Management*, **17**: 49–54.

World Health Organization (1996). *Cancer Pain Relief* (2nd edn.) World Health Organization, Geneva.

Zeppetella, G. (1999). How do terminally ill patients at home take their medication? *Palliative Medicine*, **13**: 469–475

Zeppetella, G. (2000a). Nebulized and intranasal fentanyl in the management of cancer-related breakthrough pain. *Palliative Medicine*, **14**: 57–58.

Zeppetella, G., O'Doherty, C.A., Collins, S. (2000b). Prevalence and characteristics of breakthrough pain in cancer patients admitted to a hospice. *Journal of Pain and Symptom Management*, **20**: 87–92.

Zeppetella, G., Ribeiro, M.D. (2003). Pharmacotherapy of cancer-related episodic pain. *Expert Opinion on Pharmacotherapy*, **4**: 493–502.

# Chapter 5

# Oral opioid drugs

Fiona Bailey & Ann Farley

## 5.1 Introduction

The WHO recommends the oral route for treating cancer pain (the concept of 'by mouth') (WHO 1996). However, although the oral route is generally effective in the management of background pain, it is often less effective in the management of breakthrough pain. Thus, oral opioids have a relatively delayed onset of action, which makes them less than ideal for the management of breakthrough pain. Nevertheless, oral opioids remain the cornerstone of the symptomatic management of breakthrough pain. This chapter will focus on those oral opioid preparations that are suitable for treating breakthrough pain (so-called 'normal-release', 'immediate-release', or 'short-acting' opioids).

This chapter will concentrate on opioids for moderate-to-severe pain (formerly 'strong opioids') (WHO 1996). Opioids for mild-to-moderate pain (formerly 'weak opioids') may be used to treat breakthrough pain in patients taking non-opioids (i.e. step 1 of the WHO ladder), but should not be used to treat breakthrough pain in patients taking other opioids for mild-to-moderate pain (i.e. step 2 of the WHO ladder), or opioids for moderate-to-severe pain (i.e. step 3 of the WHO ladder). There are a number of oral opioids for mild-to-moderate pain. Table 5.1 lists the relevant agents available in the United Kingdom. Tables 5.2 and 5.3 summarize basic clinical and pharmacokinetic data on these opioids.

## 5.2 Route considerations

As discussed, the oral route of administration is recommended by the WHO for treating cancer pain (WHO 1996) and is the traditional route for treating other cancer-related symptoms (Hanks *et al* 2004).

**Table 5.1** Oral opioids for mild-to-moderate pain that are available in the United Kingdom for the treatment of breakthrough pain (Anonymous 2005)

| Generic name | Trade name | Formulations | Comments |
|---|---|---|---|
| Codeine phosphate | Non-proprietary syrup | Liquid 25 mg/5 ml | POM |
| | Non-proprietary tablets | Tablet 15 mg 30 mg 60 mg | POM |
| Dihydrocodeine tartrate | Non-proprietary oral solution | Liquid 10 mg/5ml | POM |
| | Non-proprietary tablets | Tablet 30 mg | POM |
| | DF 118 Forte® tablets(Martindale) | Tablet 40 mg (100 per pack) | POM |

| Tramadol hydrochloride | Non-proprietary capsules | Capsule<br>50 mg | POM |
| | Tramake Insts® sachets<br>(Galen) | Sachet (effervescent powder)<br>50 mg<br>100 mg<br>(60 per pack) | POM.<br>50 mg sachets contain 9.7 mmol Na$^+$; 100 mg sachets contain 14.6 mmol Na$^+$. Contains aspartame.<br>Lemon flavour. |
| | Zamadol Melt® tablets<br>(Viatris) | Tablet – should be sucked and then swallowed.<br>50 mg<br>(60 per pack, 100 per pack) | POM.<br>May be dissolved in water.<br>Contains aspartame.<br>Mint flavour. |
| | Zamadol® capsules<br>(Viatris) | Capsule<br>50 mg<br>(100 per pack) | POM |
| | Zydol® soluble tablets<br>(Grünenthal) | Tablet<br>50 mg<br>(20 per pack, 100 per pack) | POM.<br>Peppermint/aniseed flavour. |
| | Zydol® capsules<br>(Grünenthal) | Capsule<br>50 mg<br>(100 per pack) | POM |

POM = Prescription-only medicine.

**Table 5.2 Basic clinical data for opioids for mild-to-moderate pain available in the United Kingdom (Thompson 1990; Twycross et al 2002; Grond & Sablotzki 2004)**

| Drug | Onset of pain relief | Time to peak pain relief | Duration of pain relief |
|------|---------------------|--------------------------|-------------------------|
| Codeine | 30–60 min | 45–60 min | 4–6 hr |
| Dihydrocodeine | 30 min | 45–60 min | 3–4 hr |
| Tramadol | 30 min | 180 min | 4–6 hr |

**Table 5.3 Basic pharmacokinetic data for opioids for mild-to-moderate pain available in the United Kingdom (Twycross et al 2002)**

| Drug | Bioavailability | Peak plasma level | Half life |
|------|----------------|-------------------|-----------|
| Codeine | 40% (range: 12–84 %) | 1–2 hr | 2.5–3.5 hr |
| Dihydrocodeine | 20% | 1.6–1.8 hr | 3–4 hr |
| Tramadol | 75% | 2 hr | 6 hr* |

\* Active metabolite has longer half life (7.4 hr).

The advantages/disadvantages of the oral route for treating breakthrough pain include (Patt & Ellison 1998; Hanks et al 2004):

Advantages
- Familiar/acceptable to patients (Walker et al 2003).
- Convenient for patients.
- Familiar/acceptable to healthcare professionals.
- Convenient for healthcare professionals.
- Large variety of oral opioid drugs available.
- Large variety of oral opioid formulations available.

Disadvantages
- Not suitable for patients with dysphagia.
- Not suitable for patients with nausea and vomiting.
- Not suitable for patients with dysfunction of the upper gastrointestinal tract.
- Variation in oral bioavailability.
- Relatively slow onset of action.
- Relatively long duration of action.

## 5.3 **Drug considerations**

### 5.3.1 **Drug**

There are a number of different oral opioids for moderate-to-severe pain. The relevant ones that are available in the United Kingdom are shown in Table 5.4. In addition some basic clinical and pharmacokinetic data on these opioids are shown in Table 5.5 and 5.6. It should be noted that although there is a significant amount of data about the pharmacokinetic profile of these opioids, there is a limited amount of data about the associated clinical effects of these opioids (e.g. time to onset of pain relief, time to maximum pain relief).

The opioid used for breakthrough pain is usually the same as the opioid used for background pain (Mercadante et al 2002). However, there is no reason why an alternative opioid cannot be used for treating breakthrough pain. Furthermore, in certain circumstances, an alternative opioid is the only option for treating breakthrough pain. For example, there is no oral preparation of fentanyl and so it is recommended that patients being treated with transdermal fentanyl use oral morphine for breakthrough pain (Table 5.7) (Anonymous 2005). Similarly, as there is no oral preparation of buprenorphine, it is recommended that patients treated with transdermal buprenorphine use sublingual buprenorphine for breakthrough pain (Anonymous 2005).

### 5.3.2 **Drug formulation**

There are a number of different formulations of oral opioids for moderate-to-severe pain. Table 5.4 lists the relevant ones available in the United Kingdom. The choice of preparation depends on a number of patient-related factors (e.g. patient preference, presence of dysphagia, presence of enteral feeding tube), and a number of drug-related factors (e.g. taste, alcohol content, sucrose content). There is little or no evidence that the formulation of the opioid affects the clinical/pharmacokinetic profile of the opioid (Figure 5.1) (Collins et al 1998).

Some of the preparations are unsuitable for use in patients with an enteral feeding tube (e.g. Palladone® [Napp Pharmaceuticals Ltd, personal communication]). Indeed, none of the oral opioid preparations is licensed/recommended by the pharmaceutical companies for use in this scenario.

In addition, some of the preparations contain alcohol which makes them unsuitable for use in patients with certain religious beliefs (e.g. Oramorph® oral solution 10 mg/5 ml). Furthermore, some patients report that the alcohol-containing preparations cause oral and/or oesophageal discomfort on ingestion. Similarly, some of the preparations contain sucrose which makes them relatively unsuitable for use in patients with diabetes mellitus (e.g. Oramorph® oral solution 10 mg/5 ml).

Table 5.4 Oral opioids for moderate-to-severe pain that are available in the United Kingdom for the treatment of breakthrough pain (Anonymous 2005)

| Generic name | Trade name | Formulations | Comments |
|---|---|---|---|
| Morphine sulphate | Oramorph® oral solution (Boehringer Ingelheim) | Colourless liquid 10 mg/5 ml (100 ml, 300 ml, 500 ml bottles) | Not a controlled drug (POM). Contains ethanol and sucrose. Discard 90 days after opening. |
| | Oramorph® concentrated oral solution (Boehringer Ingelheim) | Red liquid 20 mg/1 ml (30 ml, 120 ml bottles) | Ethanol and sucrose free. Discard 120 days after opening. |
| | Oramorph® Unit Dose Vials (Boehringer Ingelheim) | Colourless liquid 10 mg/5 ml 30 mg/5 ml 100 mg/5ml (20 per pack) | 10 mg/5 ml UDV not a controlled drug (POM). Ethanol and sucrose free. Single use. |
| | Sevredol® tablets (Napp) | Coloured tablet 10 mg – blue (marked IR 10) 20 mg – pink (marked IR 20) 50 mg – green (marked IR 50) (56 per pack) | |

| Hydromorphone hydrochloride | Palladone® capsules (Napp) | Coloured capsules 1.3 mg – orange/clear (marked HNR 1.3) 2.6 mg – red/clear (marked HNR 2.6) (56 per pack) | Capsules can be opened and contents sprinkled onto cold, soft, food if necessary. |
|---|---|---|---|
| Oxycodone hydrochloride | OxyNorm® liquid (Napp) | Colourless liquid 5 mg/5 ml (250 ml bottle) | |
| | OxyNorm® concentrate (Napp) | Orange liquid 10 mg/1 ml (120 ml bottle) | Contains sunset yellow (E110). |
| | OxyNorm® capsules (Napp) | Coloured capsules 5 mg – orange/beige (marked ONR 5) 10 mg – white/beige (marked ONR 10) 20 mg – pink/beige (marked ONR 20) (56 per pack) | 5 mg capsule contains sunset yellow (E110). |

POM = Prescription-only medicine.

**Table 5.5** Basic clinical data for opioids for moderate-to-severe pain available in the United Kingdom (Thompson, 1990; Leow et al 1992, Twycross et al 1998; Twycross et al 2002)

| Drug | Onset of pain relief | Time to peak pain relief | Duration of pain relief |
|------|---------------------|--------------------------|-------------------------|
| Morphine | 20–30 min | 60–90 min | 3–6 hr |
| Hydromorphone | 30 min | No data available | 4–5 hr |
| Oxycodone | 20–30 min | 120 min | 4–6 hr |

**Table 5.6** Basic pharmacokinetic data for opioids for moderate-to-severe pain available in the United Kingdom (Twycross et al 2002)

| Drug | Bioavailability | Peak plasma level | Half life |
|------|----------------|-------------------|-----------|
| Morphine | 35% (range: 15–64%) | 15–60 min | 1.5–4.5 hr |
| Hydromorphone | Range: 37–62% | 1 hr | 2.5 hr |
| Oxycodone | 75% (range: 60–87%) | 1–1.5 hr | 3.5 hr |

**Table 5.7** Breakthrough dose of oral morphine for background dose of transdermal fentanyl (Janssen-Cilag Ltd, data on file)

| Background dose of transdermal fentanyl (µg/hr) | Breakthrough dose of oral morphine (mg) |
|------------------------------------------------|------------------------------------------|
| 25 | <20 |
| 50 | 25–35 |
| 75 | 40–50 |
| 100 | 55–65 |
| 125 | 70–80 |
| 150 | 85–95 |
| 175 | 100–110 |
| 200 | 115–125 |
| 225 | 130–140 |
| 250 | 145–155 |
| 275 | 160–170 |
| 300 | 175–185 |

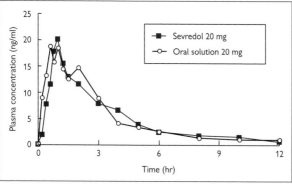

**Figure 5.1** Mean plasma morphine concentrations following oral administration of 20 mg tablet of morphine (Sevredol®) and 20 mg solution of morphine (Napp Pharmaceuticals Ltd, data on file)

### 5.3.3 **Drug dose**

The 'correct dose' of breakthrough medication is the dose that provides maximal analgesia with minimal side effects (Zeppetella & Ribeiro 2002). An Expert Working Group of the EAPC recommended using 1/6 (~ 17%) of the daily dose of background opioid analgesia (Hanks et al 2001). However, the Expert Working Group added that 'it may be that the optimal dose for breakthrough pain can only be determined by titration' (Hanks et al 2001). Other authorities have recommended using between 5–15% of the daily dose of background opioid analgesia (Cherny & Portenoy 1993).

Coluzzi et al (2001) examined the use of oral morphine for the treatment of breakthrough pain within the context of a double-blind, randomized, controlled trial of oral transmucosal fentanyl citrate. The trial showed that there was no relationship between the dose of oral morphine (or oral transmucosal fentanyl citrate) needed to control the breakthrough pain and the dose of opioid needed to control the background pain (Figures 5.2 and 5.3). Furthermore, the trial also confirmed that the time to maximum pain relief is at least 60 min after oral administration of morphine (Figure 5.4).

On the basis of the above, it would seem reasonable to initially prescribe 1/6 of the daily dose of background opioid analgesia, and then to titrate the dose upwards/downwards according to the response achieved. Thus, if the pain is not relieved and side effects are not troublesome, then the dose should be titrated upwards. In contrast, if the pain is relieved but side effects are troublesome, then the dose should be titrated downwards. Obviously, if the pain is not relieved and side effects are troublesome, then an alternative treatment should be prescribed.

## 5.4 **Drug usage**

The usefulness of oral opioids for treating breakthrough pain depends on a number of factors:

- The opioid improves the pain ('opioid-responsive'/'opioid-sensitive' pain).
- The clinical / pharmacokinetic characteristics of the opioid match the temporal characteristics of the pain.
- The patient can utilize the oral route (see above).

Unfortunately, the clinical/pharmacokinetic characteristics of oral opioids often do not match the temporal characteristics of the pains. Indeed, an Expert Working Group of the EAPC stated that oral opioids are "not suitable for pains with a short onset and duration" (Mercadante *et al* 2002). It is unclear what constitutes a 'short duration', although it is likely to be less than 30 min (i.e. the mean time to onset of pain relief for oral opioids).

The role of oral opioids in treating breakthrough pain also depends on the particular subtype of breakthrough pain:

- Spontaneous pain – oral opioids are given once the pain has begun (assuming the above criteria apply).
- Incident pain – in cases of non-volitional pain, oral opioids are given once the pain has begun. However, in cases of volitional pain or procedural pain, oral opioids can be given in advance of the precipitating event in order to try to prevent or ameliorate the incident pain. It is important that the opioids are given far enough in advance of the event. For example, in the case of oral morphine, the dose needs to be given at least 30 min (time to onset of pain relief), and probably 60 min (time to maximum pain relief) in advance of the event. The latter scenario may be the most appropriate application of the oral route of administration.
- End-of-dose failure – oral opioids can be given to relieve pain prior to modification of the background analgesic regimen.

## 5.5 **Other considerations**

### 5.5.1 **Drug acceptability**

In a survey looking at the acceptability of different routes of administration for breakthrough medication, 97% of patients stated that the oral route was acceptable for 'mild-to-moderate pain', whilst 88% of patients stated that the oral route was acceptable for 'severe pain' (see Tables 4.2 and 4.3) (Walker *et al* 2003). The only concern about the oral route was its time to onset of effect (i.e. 30 min).

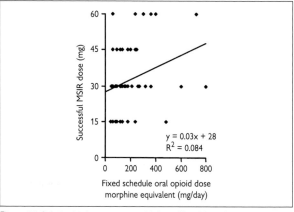

**Figure 5.2** Relationship between successful dose of breakthrough oral morphine ('MSIR') and background dose of oral opioid (reproduced with permission from Coluzzi et al 2001)

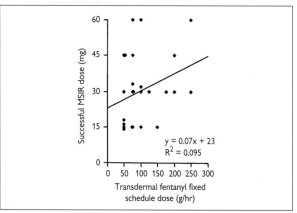

**Figure 5.3** Relationship between successful dose of breakthrough oral morphine ('MSIR') and background dose of transdermal fentanyl (reproduced with permission from Coluzzi et al 2001)

Figures 5.2 and 5.3 reproduced with permission from Coluzzi, P.H., et al. (2001). Breakthrough cancer pain: a randomized trial comparing oral transmucosal fentanyl citrate (OTFC) and morphine sulfate immediate release (MSIR). Pain, **91**: 123–130. By the International Association for the study of Pain® (IASP®).

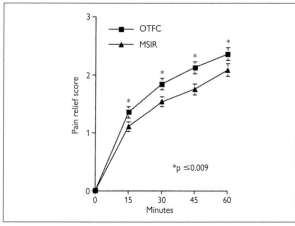

**Figure 5.4** Timing of pain relief with successful dose of breakthrough oral morphine ('MSIR') (reproduced with permission from Coluzzi *et al* 2001)

### 5.5.2 Drug costs

The oral route is considered to be relatively cost-effective (Patt & Ellison 1998). However, although oral opioids are relatively inexpensive to purchase, they will only be truly cost-effective if they actually relieve the breakthrough pain. Unrelieved breakthrough pain is associated with an increased use of healthcare services (i.e. increased outpatient visits, increased inpatient admissions) (Fortner *et al* 2002). The impact of the increased use of healthcare services is a rise in direct costs (e.g. prescription costs), and in indirect costs (e.g. transportation costs) for the health service, patient, and their carers (Fortner *et al* 2003).

## References

Anonymous (2005). British National Formulary 50. BMJ Publishing Group Ltd and Royal Pharmaceutical Society of Great Britain, London.

Cherny, N.I., Portenoy, R.K. (1993). Cancer pain management. Current strategy. *Cancer*, **72** (11 Suppl): 3393–3415.

Collins, S.L., Faura, C.C., Moore, A., McQuay, H.J. (1998). Peak plasma concentrations after oral morphine: a systematic review. *Journal of Pain and Symptom Management*, **16**: 388–402.

Figure 5.4 reproduced with permission from Coluzzi, P.H., *et al.* (2001). Breakthrough cancer pain: a randomized trial comparing oral transmucosal fentanyl citrate (OTFC) and morphine sulfate immediate release (MSIR). *Pain*, **91**: 123–130. By the International Association for the study of Pain® (IASP®).

Coluzzi, P.H., Schwartzberg, L., Conroy, Jr J.D., et al. (2001). Breakthrough cancer pain: a randomized trial comparing oral transmucosal fentanyl citrate (OTFC) and morphine sulfate immediate release (MSIR). *Pain*, **91**: 123–130.

Fortner, B.V., Demarco, G., Irving, G., et al. (2003). Description and predictors of direct and indirect costs of pain reported by cancer patients. *Journal of Pain and Symptom Management*, **25**: 9–18.

Fortner, B.V., Okon, T.A., Portenoy, R.K. (2002). A survey of pain-related hospitalizations, emergency department visits, and physician office visits reported by cancer patients with and without history of breakthrough pain. *Journal of Pain*, **3**: 38–44.

Grond, S., Sablotzki, A. (2004). Clinical pharmacology of tramadol. *Clinical Pharmacokinetics*, **43**: 879–923.

Hanks, G.W., de Conno, F., Cherny, N., et al. (2001). Morphine and alternative opioids in cancer pain: the EAPC recommendations. *British Journal of Cancer*, **84**: 587–593.

Hanks, G., Roberts, C.J., Davies, A.N. (2004). Principles of drug use in palliative medicine. In Doyle, D., Hanks, G., Cherny, N., Calman, K., ed. *Oxford Textbook of Palliative Medicine*, (3rd edn). Oxford University Press, Oxford, 213–225.

Leow, K.P., Smith, M.T., Williams, B., Cramond, T. (1992). Single-dose and steady-state pharmacokinetics and pharmacodynamics of oxycodone in patients with cancer. *Clinical Pharmacology and Therapeutics*, **52**: 487–495.

Mercadante, S., Radbruch, L., Caraceni, A., et al. (2002). Episodic (breakthrough) pain. Consensus Conference of an Expert Working Group of the European Association for Palliative Care. *Cancer*, **94**: 832–839.

Patt, R.B., Ellison, N.M. (1998). Breakthrough pain in cancer patients: characteristics, prevalence, and treatment. *Oncology (Huntington)*, **12**: 1035–1052.

Thompson, J.W. (1990). Clinical pharmacology of opioid agonists and partial agonists. In Doyle, D., ed. *Opioids in the Treatment of Cancer Pain*. Royal Society of Medicine Services Ltd, London, 17–38.

Twycross, R., Wilcock, A., Thorp, S. (1998). *Palliative Care Formulary*. Radcliffe Medical Press Ltd, Abingdon.

Twycross, R., Wilcock, A., Charlesworth, S., Dickman, A. (2002). *Palliative Care Formulary*, (2nd edn). Radcliffe Medical Press, Abingdon.

Walker, G., Wilcock, A., Manderson, C. et al. (2003). The acceptability of different routes of administration of analgesia for breakthrough pain. *Palliative Medicine*, **17**: 219–221.

World Health Organization (1996). *Cancer Pain Relief* (2nd edn) World Health Organization, Geneva.

Zeppetella, G., Ribeiro, M.D. (2002). Episodic pain in patients with advanced cancer. *American Journal of Hospice and Palliative Care*, **19**: 267–276.

# Chapter 6

# Oral transmucosal opioid drugs

Giovambattista Zeppetella

## 6.1 Introduction

The ideal treatment for breakthrough pain is an analgesic with good efficacy, a rapid onset of action and a short duration of action, and minimal adverse effects. As discussed in Chapter 5, the oral route may not be suitable for many patients with breakthrough pain. Thus the pharmacokinetic profile of many orally delivered drugs does not closely mirror the characteristics of breakthrough pain, resulting in only partially effective treatment and/or troublesome adverse effects. In an effort to deliver more effective treatment, various other routes of administration have been explored including the transmucosal routes of administration. The transmucosal routes include ocular, nasal, buccal, sublingual, pulmonary, rectal, and vaginal. This chapter will outline the role of the oral transmucosal routes (buccal, sublingual), whilst Chapter 7 will outline the role of certain other transmucosal routes (nasal, pulmonary, rectal), in the management of breakthrough pain.

## 6.2 Oral mucosa

The oral mucosa refers to the lining of the oral cavity. It is composed of an outer layer of stratified squamous epithelium, below which lies the basement membrane, and then the lamina propria (connective tissue layer). The total surface area of the oral mucosa is ~200 cm$^2$, which is relatively small compared to the gastrointestinal tract (~350 000 cm$^2$) (Zhang *et al* 2002). The lamina propria is highly vascularized and drugs diffusing into the oral mucosa have access to the systemic circulation via its capillaries and venous drainage (via the internal jugular vein). The rate of blood flow through the oral mucosa is substantial; rates are 0.97 ml/min/cm$^2$ in the sublingual mucosa and 2.4 ml/min/cm$^2$ in the buccal mucosa. The oral mucosa is covered by a layer of saliva, which is secreted by the three pairs of major salivary glands (parotid, submandibular, sublingual) and the hundreds of minor salivary glands distributed throughout the mouth.

The composition of the epithelium varies depending on the site within the oral cavity. For example, the hard palate, the gingivae, and the dorsal surface of the tongue are covered by a layer of keratinized cells, whilst the epithelium covering the soft palate, the buccal mucosa and the sublingual mucosa is non-keratinized. (Non-keratinized epithelium is more permeable to water than keratinized epithelium.) Similarly, the thickness of the epithelium varies according to the site: for example, the buccal mucosa is approximately 3 times as thick as the sublingual mucosa: (500–600 μm versus 100–200 μm) (Lee 2001). As a result of these characteristics, the permeability of the sublingual mucosa is greater than that of the buccal mucosa, which is greater than that of the remainder of the oral mucosa (Shojaei 1998).

The absorption of drugs across the oral mucosa involves a process of passive absorption, and may involve the transcellular or the paracellular route (via the intercellular spaces), or a combination of the two (Hao & Hang 2003). Lipophilic drugs are predominantly absorbed using the transcellular route, whilst hydrophilic drugs are predominantly absorbed via the paracellular route. It should be noted that lipophilic drugs need to also have a degree of hydrophilicity in order to traverse the inner part of the cell (Zhang et al 2002). Paracellular absorption is limited by the small surface area available for this type of absorption (Hao & Hang 2003).

A number of drug factors affect the absorption of drugs across the oral mucosa, including the lipophilicity of the drug (see above), the ionized fraction of the drug (ionized drugs are less permeable), and the duration of contact with the mucosa (Hao & Hang 2003). The amount of drug that can be absorbed is small, and so only potent drugs are suitable for oral transmucosal administration (Zhang et al 2002).

Patients with oral mucosal disease may have altered oral transmucosal absorption (Hao & Hang 2003). Indeed, patients may have either decreased absorption of drugs (mucosal thickening), or increased absorption of drugs (muscal inflammation). Similarly, patients with salivary gland dysfuntion may have altered oral transmucosal absorption. Thus saliva is important in maintaining the pH of the oral cavity, which can affect the ionized fraction of the drug. Moreover, saliva may be necessary to dissolve the drug formulation (tablets, lozenges).

## 6.3 **Oral transmucosal administration**

The oral transmucosal route offers several advantages over the gastrointestinal tract and other alternative routes of administration (Zhang et al 2002):

- Acceptable to patients (non-invasive) (Walker et al 2003).
- Convenient for patient.
- Convenient for healthcare professionals.

- Suitable for patients with dysphagia.
- Suitable for patients with nausea and vomiting.
- Suitable for patients with dysfunction of the upper gastrointestinal tract.
- Potentially fast onset of action.
- Avoidance of degradation by gastric acid/enzymes.
- Avoidance of first-pass metabolism by liver enzymes.

Oral transmucosal drug delivery does not require expertise, preparation, technical equipment or patient supervision. Thus, oral transmucosal administration is convenient for patients, convenient for healthcare professionals, and is more cost effective than certain other (invasive) routes of administration (Zhang et al 2002). Furthermore, oral transmucosal administration of certain drugs can provide patients with an onset of action approaching that seen with intravenous administration.

The disadvantages of the oral transmucosal route include (Zhang et al 2002):

- Not suitable for patients with dryness of mouth.
- Not suitable for patients with oral pathology.
- Limited number of suitable drugs.
- Limited number of suitable formulations.
- Variation in oral transmucosal bioavailability.

## 6.4 Opioids approved for oral transmucosal administration

Currently, the two drugs licensed for administration using the oral transmucosal route in the United Kingdom are oral transmucosal fentanyl citrate (buccal administration) and buprenorphine (sublingual administration) (Anonymous 2005). A variety of other opioids have been subject to oral transmucosal administration. However, many of these opioids are not very lipophilic and, therefore, not suited for buccal or sublingual administration. Figure 6.1 shows the percentage absorption for selected opioids administered by the sublingual route (Weinberg et al 1988).

### 6.4.1 Fentanyl

#### 6.4.1.1 Drug characteristics

Fentanyl is a synthetic opioid and an agonist at the μ receptor (analgesic effect).

#### 6.4.1.2 Product characteristics

In the United Kingdom, fentanyl is available as a lozenge (Actiq®: doses – 200 μg, 400 μg, 600 μg, 800 μg, 1200 μg, 1600 μg) as well as a transdermal patch and a parenteral preparation (Anonymous 2005).

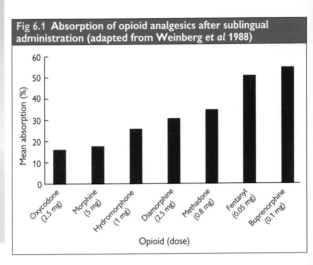

Fig 6.1 **Absorption of opioid analgesics after sublingual administration (adapted from Weinberg et al 1988)**

Opioid (dose)

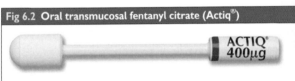

Fig 6.2 **Oral transmucosal fentanyl citrate (Actiq®)**

The lozenge (oral transmucosal fentanyl citrate) is licensed for the management of breakthrough pain in patients already receiving opioid therapy for chronic cancer pain (Anonymous 2005).

Oral transmucosal fentanyl citrate (OTFC) consists of a hardened, sweetened, fentanyl-impregnated lozenge on a plastic handle (Figure 6.2). OTFC is rubbed against the inside of the cheek, which allows the lozenge to be dissolved by the saliva and the fentanyl to be absorbed through the buccal mucosa.

It takes ~15 min to dissolve the lozenge. However, patients with a dry mouth may take longer/be unable to dissolve the lozenge. It is recommended that the lozenge be removed from the mouth if the pain is relieved before the lozenge has completely dissolved; the partly consumed lozenge should not be recycled, but should be dissolved under hot running water.

A number of pharmaceutical companies are developing alternative oral transmucosal preparations of fentanyl for the management of breakthrough pain, including various sublingual sprays and a buccal/sublingual effervescent tablet. In addition, several authors have reported success with the sublingual administration of the parenteral preparation of fentanyl (Gardner-Nix 2001; Zeppetella 2001; Duncan 2002).

### 6.4.1.3 Pharmacokinetic profile
Fentanyl is highly lipid-soluble and 80% non-ionized, making it ideally suited for transmucosal absorption. The bioavailability of OTFC is 50%: 25% is rapidly absorbed through the buccal mucosa, whilst 25% is more slowly absorbed through the gastrointestinal mucosa as a result of swallowing the drug (Hanks 2001).

### 6.4.1.4 Clinical data
OTFC can provide pain relief within 5–10 min, with the peak effect occurring within 20–30 min (Hanks 2001). The rapid onset of action is dependent on absorption through the buccal mucosa. Indeed, patients who suck the lozenge rather than rub the lozenge against the inside of their cheek will experience a delayed/reduced effect. The duration of analgesia is ~2 hr (Hanks 2001).

There have been numerous studies of the use of OTFC in the management of cancer-related breakthrough pain (Mystakidou et al 2005). Table 6.1 shows data from the randomized trials of OTFC (Christie et al 1998; Farrar et al 1998; Portenoy et al 1999; Coluzzi et al 2001). In general, OTFC is effective in treating breakthrough pain (Figures 6.3 and 6.4), and well tolerated by this group of patients.

The randomized trials have demonstrated that there is no correlation between the dose of opioid needed to control the background pain and the dose of OTFC needed to control the breakthrough pain (Figures 6.5 and 6.6) (Christie et al 1998; Portenoy et al 1999; Coluzzi et al 2001). In other words, the dose of OTFC requires individual titration. Figure 6.7 shows the conventional titration schedule for OTFC (Zeppetella 2005). However, more rapid titration schedules have been developed, and are presently being tested (Zeppetella 2005).

The side effects of OTFC are typical of other opioid preparations and include somnolence, nausea, vomiting, and dizziness (Christie et al 1998; Farrar et al 1998; Portenoy et al 1999; Coluzzi et al 2001). It should be noted that some patients are unable to use OTFC, including patients that are severely disabled (and cannot agitate the preparation), that are severely fatigued (and cannot agitate the preparation), that have ongoing oral dryness (and cannot dissolve the preparation), and that have ongoing oral pathology (that may affect absorption of the preparation).

Dry mouth is one of the main reasons cited for not being able to use OTFC. However, it is usually possible to treat this condition. Moreover, treatment of the dry mouth may allow treatment of breakthrough pain with OTFC (Davies & Vriens 2005).

**Table 6.1a Randomized trials of oral transmucosal fentanyl citrate**

| Study | Methodology | Principal outcomes |
|---|---|---|
| Christie et al (1998) | Multicentre, double-blind, randomized, dose-titration study of OTFC. 62 cancer patients using transdermal fentanyl for background analgesia. | • 76% patients titrated to an effective dose of OTFC. <br>• No relationship was found between the successful dose of OTFC and the dose of background transdermal fentanyl. <br>• OTFC produced significantly quicker/better pain relief than usual breakthrough analgesic. <br>• Global satisfaction significantly higher for OTFC than usual breakthrough analgesic. <br>• The most common adverse effects of OTFC were somnolence, nausea, dizziness, and vomiting. |
| Portenoy et al (1999) | Multicentre, double-blind, randomized dose-titration study of OTFC. 65 cancer patients using oral opioids for background analgesia. | • 74% patients titrated to an effective dose of OTFC. <br>• No relationship was found between the successful dose of OTFC and the dose of background oral opioid. <br>• OTFC produced significantly quicker/better pain relief than usual breakthrough analgesic. <br>• Global satisfaction significantly higher for OTFC than usual breakthrough analgesic. <br>• The most common adverse effects of OTFC were somnolence, dizziness, nausea and headache. |

OTFC = oral transmucosal fentanyl citrate

**Table 6.1b Randomized trials of oral transmucosal fentanyl citrate**

| Study | Methodology | Principal outcomes |
|-------|-------------|--------------------|
| Farrar et al 1998 | Multicentre, double-blind, randomized, controlled, crossover trial of OTFC versus placebo. 92 cancer patients using oral opioids or transdermal fentanyl for background analgesia. Patients only eligible for main trial if they responded to OTFC. | • OTFC produced significantly quicker/better pain relief than placebo.<br>• Global performance of OTFC better than placebo.<br>• Patients required significantly less additional rescue medication when using OTFC.<br>• Most patients chose to continue with OTFC following the trial.<br>• The most common adverse effects of OTFC were dizziness, nausea, somnolence, constipation, and asthenia. |
| Coluzzi et al, 2001 | Multicentre, double-blind, randomized, controlled, crossover trial of OTFC versus oral morphine. 93 cancer patients using oral opioids or transdermal opioid for background analgesia. Patients only eligible for main trial if they responded to OTFC. | • No relationship was found between the successful dose of OTFC and the dose of background oral opioid or transdermal opioid (Figure 6.5 and 6.6).<br>• OTFC produced significantly quicker/better pain relief than oral morphine (Figure 6.3 & 6.4).<br>• Global performance of OTFC better than placebo.<br>• Most patients chose to continue with OTFC following the trial.<br>• The most common adverse effects of OTFC were somnolence, nausea, constipation, and dizziness. |

OTFC = oral transmucosal fentanyl citrate.

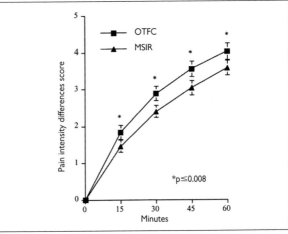

**Figure 6.3** Pain intensity difference scores with oral transmucosal fentanyl citrate (OTFC) and immediate-release oral morphine sulphate (MSIR) (reproduced with permission from Coluzzi *et al* 2001)

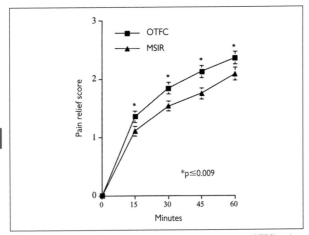

**Figure 6.4** Pain-relief scores with oral transmucosal fentanyl citrate (OTFC) and immediate-release oral morphine sulphate (MSIR) (reproduced with permission from Coluzzi *et al* 2001)

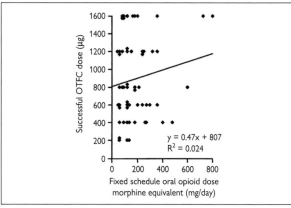

**Figure 6.5** Relationship between successful dose of oral transmucosal fentanyl citrate (OTFC) and background dose of oral opioid (reproduced with permission from Coluzzi *et al* 2001)

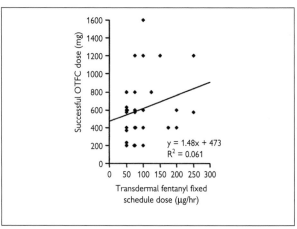

**Figure 6.6** Relationship between successful dose of oral transmucosal fentanyl citrate (OTFC) and background dose of transdermal fentanyl (reproduced with permission from Coluzzi *et al* 2001)

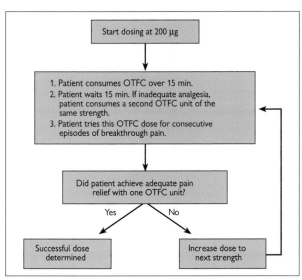

**Figure 6.7** Conventional titration scheme for oral transmucosal fentanyl citrate (adapted from Zeppetella 2005)

### 6.4.2 Buprenorphine

#### 6.4.2.1 Drug characteristics

Buprenorphine is a semi-synthetic opioid, and is a partial agonist at the μ-receptor (analgesic effect).

#### 6.4.2.2 Product characteristics

In the United Kingdom, buprenorphine is available as a sublingual tablet (Temgesic®: doses – 200 µg, 400 µg), as well as a transdermal patch and a parenteral preparation (Anonymous 2005). The sublingual tablet is licensed for the management of moderate to severe pain; the sublingual tablet is primarily used in the management of background pain, but is also recommended for use in the management of breakthrough pain in patients prescribed the transdermal patch (Anonymous 2005).

#### 6.4.2.3 Pharmacokinetic profile

Buprenorphine is highly lipophilic, and is well absorbed across mucosal membranes. The percentage absorption is ~55% after sublingual administration (Figure 6.1) (Weinberg et al 1988), although it is somewhat less after buccal administration (Davis 2005). However, the rate of systemic absorption can be slow: peak plasma concentrations occur 0.5–3 hr after sublingual administration (Davis, 2005).

### 6.4.2.4 *Clinical data*

The reported onset of action of sublingual buprenorphine is ~15–30 min, the peak analgesic effect occurs at ~60–120 min, and the duration of action is ~8 hr (Thompson 1990). (The delayed peak analgesic effect and the long duration of action are disadvantageous for the treatment of breakthrough pain.)

There have been numerous studies of the use of sublingual buprenorphine in the management of cancer-related pain (Davis 2005). The majority of these studies report its use for background pain, but some also report its use for breakthrough pain (with the transdermal buprenorphine patch) (Sittl *et al* 2003; Sorge & Sittl 2004). However, there appear to have been no studies of the specific use of sublingual buprenorphine in the management of cancer-related breakthrough pain.

The adverse effects encountered with buprenorphine are typical of those encountered with opioid analgesics. Buprenorphine is reported to cause more dizziness, nausea and vomiting than morphine (Davis 2005). However, it is reported to cause less respiratory depression and constipation than morphine (Davis 2005). It should be noted that the effects of buprenorphine are only partially reversed by opioid antagonists (e.g. naloxone) (Anonymous 2005).

## 6.5 Other opioids for oral transmucosal administration

### 6.5.1 Morphine

Morphine is not very lipophilic and 90% of its molecules are ionized at the normal oral pH (Coluzzi 1998). Thus, the physicochemical properties of morphine are not favourable for oral transmucosal absorption. Indeed, the percentage absorption is only 18% after sublingual administration (Figure 6.1) (Weinberg *et al* 1988). In addition, the time to maximum peak concentration and the maxmimum peak concentration are reported to be similar for the sublingual and the oral routes (McQuay *et al* 1986).

Efficacy studies appear to be contradictory. However, a review of the literature on the use of sublingual morphine stated that 'the limited clinical data do not provide compelling evidence for the effectiveness of sublingual morphine for the rapid relief of pain in cancer patients' (Coluzzi 1998). Nevertheless, sublingual administration of morphine may have a more general role to play in patients unable to use the oral and /or the parenteral routes (Coluzzi 1998).

### 6.5.2 Diamorphine

Diamorphine is a semi-synthetic analogue of morphine. It is much more lipophilic than morphine. The percentage absorption is ~30% after sublingual absorption (see Figure 6.1) (Weinberg *et al* 1988).

Sublingual diamorphine has been reported to be effective in the management of pain in adults (McQuay *et al* 1986). Similarly, buccal diamorphine has been found to be useful in the management of breakthrough pain in children (Dr Finella Craig, personal communication). However, there does not appear to have been a formal investigation of the use of oral transmucosal diamorphine in the management of breakthrough pain. Nevertheless intranasal (transmucosal) diamorphine may be useful in the management of breakthrough pain (Kendall *et al* 2003).

In spite of the above, diamorphine is not ideally suited for the treatment of breakthrough pain, since the four-hourly duration of action will outlast the duration of most breakthrough pains.

### 6.5.3 **Hydromorphone**

Hydromorphone has a relatively low lipid solubility, which results in limited transmucosal absorption (Figure 6.1) (Weinberg *et al* 1988). The low bioavailability and long duration of action of hydromorphone (~4 hr) mean that this drug is not ideally suited for the treatment of breakthrough pain.

### 6.5.4 **Oxycodone**

Oxycodone has a very low lipid solubility, which results in very limited transmucosal absorption (Figure 6.1) (Weinberg *et al* 1988). Again, the low bioavailability and long duration of action of transmucosal oxycodone (~4 hr) mean that this drug is not ideally suited for the treatment of breakthrough pain. Nevertheless, there are reports of buccal administration of oxycodone in the management of background pain (Parodi *et al* 1997).

### 6.5.5 **Methadone**

Methadone is a lipophilic drug, which is well absorbed across mucosal membranes. The percentage absorption is 35% after sublingual administration (Figure 6.1) (Weinberg *et al* 1988). The sublingual bioavailability is reported to be similar to the oral bioavailability (McQuay *et al* 1986). In addition, the time to maximum peak concentration and the maximum peak concentration are reported to be similar for the two routes (McQuay *et al* 1986).

Sublingual methadone has been reported to be effective in the management of pain in adults (McQuay *et al* 1986). In view of the comparable pharmacokinetic profile of oral and sublingual methadone (McQuay *et al* 1986), it would seem reasonable to suppose that the clinical profile is similar for sublingual and oral methadone. Oral methadone is reported to have an onset of action of 30–60 min, a peak analgesic effect at 30–120 min, and a duration of action of 6–8 hr (Thompson 1990). However, a recent study of oral methadone for breakthrough pain stated that some patients reported an analgesic effect at 10 min following ingestion of the oral methadone (Fisher *et al* 2004).

The fast onset of action of sublingual methadone would be advantageous, although the pharmacokinetics of methadone may be problematic, in the management of breakthrough pain.

### 6.5.6 **Alfentanil**

Alfentanil is a synthetic opioid analgesic that is chemically similar to fentanyl. It is less lipophilic than fentanyl, but has a more rapid onset of action and shorter duration of action when given parenterally (Scholz et al 1996). For example, when given intravenously, the onset of action is <2 min, and the duration of action is 10 min (Twycross et al 2002). These characteristics suggest that alfentanil could be particularly helpful in the management of breakthrough pain.

A parenteral preparation of alfentanil has been reported to be effective and well tolerated when administered buccally/sublingually in a small case series of patients with cancer-related breakthrough pain (Duncan 2002). Interestingly, patients preferred buccal administration of the preparation. It should be noted that the main reason for choosing alfentanil in this series was the availability of a suitable (concentrated) preparation of alfentanil, i.e. only small volumes of alfentanil were required to be administered.

### 6.5.7 **Sufentanil**

Sufentanil is another synthetic opioid analgesic, which is chemically similar to fentanyl. It is more lipophilic than fentanyl, and has a more rapid onset of action and shorter duration of action when given parenterally (Scholz et al 1996). Again, these characteristics suggest that sufentanil could be particularly helpful in the management of breakthrough pain.

There have been a number of published reports supporting the role of sublingual sufentanil in the management of breakthrough pain (Kunz et al 1993; Gardner-Nix 2001). In the study by Gardner Nix, the onset of action was reported to be between 4–6 min, and the duration of action 35 min (Gardner-Nix 2001). Indeed, some patients required a combination of the short acting sufentanil and a longer acting oral opioid (morphine, hydromorphone) to control some longer lasting episodes of breakthrough pain. Again, the main reason for choosing sufentanil in this series was the availability of a suitable (concentrated) preparation of sufentanil.

## References

Anonymous (2005). *British National Formulary 50*. BMJ Publishing Group Ltd and Royal Pharmaceutical Society of Great Britain, London.

Christie, J.M., Simmonds, M., Patt, R. et al. (1998). Dose-titration, multicenter study of oral transmucosal fentanyl citrate for the treatment of breakthrough pain in cancer patients using transdermal fentanyl for persistent pain. *Journal of Clinical Oncology*, **16**: 3238–3245.

Coluzzi, P.H. (1998). Sublingual morphine: efficacy reviewed. *Journal of Pain and Symptom Management*, **16**: 184–192.

Coluzzi, P.H., Schwartzberg, L., Conroy, Jr. J.D. *et al.* (2001). Breakthrough cancer pain: a randomized trial comparing oral transmucosal fentanyl citrate (OTFC) and morphine sulfate immediate release (MSIR). *Pain*, **91**: 123–130.

Davies, A.N., Vriens, J. (2005). Oral transmucosal fentanyl citrate and xerostomia (dry mouth). *Journal of Pain and Symptom Management*, **30**: 496–497.

Davis, M.P. (2005). Buprenorphine in cancer pain. *Supportive Care in Cancer*, **13**: 878–887.

Duncan, A. (2002). The use of fentanyl and alfentanil sprays for episodic pain. *Palliative Medicine*, **16**: 550.

Farrar, J.T., Cleary, J., Rauck, R., *et al.* (1998). Oral transmucosal fentanyl citrate: randomized, double-blinded, placebo-controlled trial for treatment of breakthrough pain in cancer patients. *Journal of the National Cancer Institute*, **90**: 611–616.

Fisher, K., Stiles, C., Hagen, N.A. (2004). Characterization of the early pharmacodynamic profile of oral methadone for cancer-related breakthrough pain: a pilot study. *Journal of Pain and Symptom Management*, **28**: 619–625.

Gardner-Nix, J. (2001). Oral transmucosal fentanyl and sufentanil for incident pain. *Journal of Pain and Symptom Management*, **22**: 627–630.

Hanks, G. (2001). Oral transmucosal fentanyl citrate for the management of breakthrough pain. *European Journal of Palliative Care*, **8**: 6–9.

Hao, J., Heng, P.W. (2003). Buccal delivery systems. *Drug Development and Industrial Pharmacy*, **29**: 821–832.

Kendal, C.E., Davies, A.N., Forbes, K. (2003). Nasal diamorphine for "breakthrough pain" in palliative care – a promising approach to a difficult problem (Abstract 509). In *Proceedings of 8th Congress of the European Association for Palliative Care.* 2–5th April, Hague, Netherlands, 92.

Kunz, K.M., Theisen, J.A., Schroeder, M.E. (1993). Severe episodic pain: management with sublingual sufentanil. *Journal of Pain and Symptom Management*, **8**: 189.

Lee, V.H. (2001). Mucosal drug delivery. *Journal of the National Cancer Institute, Monographs*, **29**: 41–44.

McQuay, H.J., Moore, R.A., Bullingham, R.E. (1986). Sublingual morphine, heroin, methadone and buprenorphine: kinetics and effects. In Foley, K.M., Inturrisi, C.E., ed. *Opioid Analgesics in the Management of Clinical Pain. Advances in Pain Research and Therapy.* Volume 8. Raven Press, New York, 407–412.

Mystakidou, K., Katsouda, E., Parpa, E., *et al.* (2005). Oral transmucosal fentanyl citrate for the treatment of breakthrough pain in cancer patients: an overview of its pharmacological and clinical characteristics. *American Journal of Hospice and Palliative Medicine*, **22**: 228–232.

Parodi, B., Russo, E., Caviglioli, G., *et al.* (1997). Buccoadhesive oxycodone hydrochloride disks: plasma pharmacokinetics in healthy volunteers and clinical study. *European Journal of Pharmaceutics and Biopharmaceutics*, **44**: 137–142.

Portenoy, R.K., Payne, R., Coluzzi, P. *et al.* (1999). Oral transmucosal fentanyl citrate (OTFC) for the treatment of breakthrough pain in cancer patients: a controlled dose titration study. *Pain*, **79**: 303–312.

Scholz, J., Steinfath, M., Schulz, M. (1996). Clinical pharmacokinetics of alfentanil, fentanyl and sufentanil. An update. *Clinical Pharmacokinetics*, **31**: 275–292.

Shojaei, A.H. (1998). Buccal mucosa as a route for systemic drug delivery: a review. *Journal of Pharmacy and Pharmaceutical Sciences*, **1**: 15–30.

Sittl, R., Griessinger, N., Likar, R. (2003). Analgesic efficacy and tolerability of transdermal buprenorphine in patients with inadequately controlled chronic pain related to cancer and other disorders: a multicenter, randomized, double-blind, placebo-controlled trial. *Clinical Therapeutics*, **25**: 150–168.

Sorge, J., Sittl, R. (2004). Transdermal buprenorphine in the treatment of chronic pain: results of a phase III, multicenter, randomized, double-blind, placebo-controlled study. *Clinical Therapeutics*, **26**: 1808–1820.

Thompson, J.W. (1990). Clinical pharmacology of opioid agonists and partial agonists. In Doyle, D., ed. *Opioids in the Treatment of Cancer Pain*. Royal Society of Medicine Services Ltd, London, 17–38.

Twycross, R., Wilcock, A., Charlesworth, S., Dickman, A. (2002). *Palliative Care Formulary*, (2nd edn.) Radcliffe Medical Press, Abingdon.

Walker, G., Wilcock, A., Manderson, C., *et al.* (2003). The acceptability of different routes of administration of analgesia for breakthrough pain. *Palliative Medicine*, **17**: 219–221.

Weinberg, D.S., Inturrisi, C.E., Reidenberg, B. *et al.* (1988). Sublingual absorption of selected opioid analgesics. *Clinical Pharmacology and Therapeutics*, **44**: 335–342.

Zeppetella, G. (2001). Sublingual fentanyl citrate for cancer-related breakthrough pain: a pilot study. *Palliative Medicine*, **15**: 323–328.

Zeppetella, J. (2005). Is the recommended titration schedule for OTFC too conservative? *European Journal of Palliative Care*, **12** (Suppl): 6–7.

Zhang, H., Zhang, J., Streisand, J.B. (2002). Oral mucosal drug delivery: clinical pharmacokinetics and therapeutic applications. *Clinical Pharmacokinetics*, **41**: 661–680.

# Chapter 7

# Opioid drugs via other routes

Ola Dale

## 7.1 Introduction

Ideally, breakthrough pain should be treated with a self-manageable method that consistently provides a rapid onset of action, good efficacy, a short duration of action, and good tolerability. Furthermore, the method must be acceptable to patients and affordable for the healthcare system.

The majority of patients with breakthrough pain are treated with oral opioids. However, as discussed in Chapter 5, the oral route of administration is not ideally suited to the treatment of breakthrough pain. Furthermore, there are a number of relative contraindications to the oral route of administration (e.g. dysphagia, nausea and vomiting).

Opioids can be delivered via a number of other routes, including rectal, intravenous, intramuscular, subcutaneous, transdermal, oral transmucosal, intranasal, and intrapulmonary routes (Stevens & Ghazi 2000). Some of these routes are regularly used to manage breakthrough pain (e.g. subcutaneous, oral transmucosal), whilst others are still being investigated for their ability to manage breakthrough pain (e.g. intranasal, intrapulmonary).

The suitability of different opioids to be delivered by different routes depends on a number of physicochemical factors (i.e. drug factors), and pharmaceutical factors (i.e. product factors). For example, methadone is not ideally suited to intranasal administration, because it causes irritation of the nasal mucosa (Dale *et al* 2002b). Similarly, fentanyl is not ideally suited to intranasal administration, because it is currently not available in a concentrated solution (Duncan 2002).

## 7.2 Enteral routes

### 7.2.1 Oral administration

A comprehensive discussion of oral administration can be found in Chapter 5. However, some comparative aspects of oral administration are shown in Table 7.1.

### 7.2.2 Rectal administration

The rectum is ~15–19 cm in length and has a surface area of ~ 200–400 cm$^2$ available for drug absorption. The upper part of the rectum drains into the portal vein, whilst the lower part of the rectum drains into the inferior vena cava (and thus circumvents the liver/first-pass metabolism). However, there are anastomoses between the two venous systems (van Hoogdalem et al 1991; Warren 1996).

Drug transport across the rectal mucosa is predominantly by passive diffusion. Hence, absorption is dependent on the extent/duration of contact of the drug with the rectal mucosa. Stool in the rectum may restrict the absorption of the drug. Furthermore, defaecation will also restrict the absorption of the drug, and reflex expulsion will occur if significant volumes are instilled/inserted into the rectum (i.e. 10–25 ml) (van Hoogdalem et al 1991; Warren, 1996). Uptake of drug from the rectum also depends to a high degree on the formulation used (e.g. liquid enemas tend to be more rapidly absorbed than solid suppositories).

Rectal administration may result in a faster onset of action than oral administration due to the time taken for the drug to reach the site of absorption for the oral route (i.e. small bowel). Indeed, it has been shown that there is more rapid uptake of methadone after rectal administration in healthy volunteers (Dale et al 2004). In addition, rectal administration may result in a higher bioavailability than oral administration for opioids that undergo extensive first-pass metabolism (e.g. morphine). However, rectal bioavailability can be extremely variable, for the reasons discussed above (Hanks et al 2004).

The rectal route has been suggested as being suitable for the treatment of breakthrough pain, although there appears to be no specific studies of the use of the rectal route for the treatment of breakthrough pain (Mercadante et al 2002). Rectal administration may be an alternative to the oral route in patients with nausea, vomiting, dysphagia, malabsorption, and bowel obstruction. It may also be an alternative to the parenteral routes in patients with bleeding disorders and immunologic deficiencies (Mercadante & Fulfaro 1999).

**Table 7.1 Characteristics of different routes of administration**

| Characteristic | Oral route | Rectal route | Intravenous route | Intramuscular route | Subcutaneous route | Transmucosal routes* | Intrapulmonary route |
|---|---|---|---|---|---|---|---|
| First-pass metabolism | ++ | (+) | – | – | – | – | – |
| Bioavailability | Variable | Variable | Maximum | High | Medium to high | Medium to high | Medium to high |
| Onset of action | 30 min | 30 min | 5 min | 10 min | 10 min | 10 min | 5 min |
| Invasive method | – | – | + | + | + | – | – |
| Self-administered method | + | + | – | – | + | + | + |
| Duration of usage | Unlimited | Medium term | Long term | Short term | Long term | ? | ? |

Oral transmucosal, intranasal

– = negative

+ = positive

The rectal route is simple, does not require any equipment, and can be used by both patients and their non-professional caregivers (Hanks *et al* 2004). However, the rectal route may be inappropriate in patients with local disease of the rectum, and may be difficult to use in patients that are very unwell/uncooperative. In addition, many patients do not find the rectal route an acceptable route of administration for drugs. For example, in the study by Walker *et al* (2003) only 24% of patients thought that the rectal route was acceptable for pain that was mild to moderate in nature, and only 48% thought that the rectal route was acceptable for pain that was severe in nature. A variety of different reasons were given for not wanting to use this route (See Table 4.2).

## 7.3  **Parenteral routes**

### 7.3.1  **Intravenous administration**

The intravenous route is associated with a 100% bioavailability (by definition), and a very rapid onset of action (~ 5 min).

Mercadante *et al* (2004) reported on the use of intravenous morphine to treat breakthrough pain episodes in patients receiving oral morphine. Intravenous morphine was found to be effective, to be well tolerated, and to be safe (in the inpatient setting). In addition, other authors have reported on the use of intravenous morphine to treat breakthrough pain episodes in patients receiving continuous infusions of morphine (i.e. intravenous patient-controlled analgesia [PCA]) (Wagner *et al* 1989; Swanson *et al* 1989).

The intravenous route requires appropriate venous access, some basic equipment (for bolus injections), and some training in performing the technique. In theory, this route can be used in community settings, and the technique can be taught to patients and their caregivers. However, in practice, this route is generally restricted to inpatient settings. It should be noted that intravenous PCA has been successfully used in community settings (Wagner *et al* 1989; Swanson *et al* 1989).

Intravenous administration has low acceptability when the pain is mild to moderate in intensity (38% acceptability), but has a higher acceptability when the pain is severe in intensity (83% acceptability) (Walker *et al* 2003). The main objections to the use of this route were dislike of injections and previous bad experiences with this route.

### 7.3.2  **Intramuscular administration**

The intramuscular route of administration is not recommended for the treatment of breakthrough pain, because of the discomfort associated with intramuscular injection (Mercadante *et al* 2002). Indeed, the intramuscular route of administration is not acceptable to many patients because of their dislike for injections (and particularly intramuscular injections) (Walker *et al* 2003). Nevertheless, in certain circumstances, there may be no alternative to the intramuscular route of administration (Hanks *et al* 2004).

### 7.3.3 Subcutaneous administration

The subcutaneous route is the most commonly used parenteral route of administration in palliative care (Hanks *et al* 2004). The subcutaneous route associated with a relatively high bioavailability: for example, a pharmacokinetic study in healthy volunteers showed that subcutaneous morphine has a bioavailability of 80–100% (higher for continuous infusion than for bolus doses) (Stuart-Harris *et al* 2000). The subcutaneous route is also associated with a relatively rapid onset of action (~10 min).

Enting *et al* (2005) reported on the use of subcutaneous hydromorphone to treat breakthrough pain: the hydromorphone was delivered using a 'pain pen' (an adapted insulin injection pen). Other studies are being planned to confirm the efficacy, tolerability, and safety of this approach. In addition, other authors have reported on the use of subcutaneous morphine to treat breakthrough pain episodes in patients receiving continuous infusions of morphine (i.e. subcutaneous PCA) (Wagner *et al* 1989; Swanson *et al* 1989).

The subcutaneous route requires some basic equipment (for bolus injections), and some training in performing the technique. It is used in community settings, and the technique can be taught to patients and carers. It should be noted that the pain pen and the subcutaneous PCA have been successfully used in community settings (Wagner *et al* 1989; Swanson *et al* 1989).

Subcutaneous administration has reasonable acceptability when the pain is mild to moderate in intensity (52% acceptability), but has a higher acceptability when the pain is severe in intensity (87% acceptability) (Walker *et al* 2003). The main objection to the use of this route was dislike of injections.

### 7.3.4 Transdermal administration

Currently, transdermal administration has no role to play in the treatment of breakthrough pain. However, new patch technology (iontophoretic technology) may alter the current state of affairs (see below).

A fentanyl hydrochloride patient-activated transdermal system (PATS) has recently been developed/approved for the treatment of postoperative pain. The system uses a low-intensity direct current to transport fentanyl from the reservoir in the patch into the subcutaneous tissues (and thence into the systemic circulation) (Sinatra 2005). The system is patient activated, delivers a 40 µg bolus of fentanyl over 10 min, and has a 10 min 'lock out' facility; the system is operational for 24 hr, and delivers a maximum of 80 boluses of fentanyl. The system compared favourably to conventional PCA in a study of postoperative pain (Viscusi *et al* 2004).

## 7.4 'Partial' parenteral routes

The partial parenteral routes include the oral transmucosal route, the intranasal route, and the intrapulmonary/inhalational route. The majority of the dispensed drug is absorbed parenterally although some of the drug is absorbed enterally as a result of unintentional swallowing.

### 7.4.1 Oral transmucosal administration

A comprehensive discussion of oral transmucosal administration can be found in Chapter 6. However, some comparative aspects of oral transmucosal administration are shown in Table 7.1.

### 7.4.2 Intranasal administration

The nose has a relatively small surface area for absorption (~ 150–180 cm$^2$). However, the nasal epithelium is highly permeable and also highly perfused with blood. The latter factors help to facilitate the absorption of drugs. A special feature of the nose is its close connection to the brain in the olfactory area (i.e. an absence of the normal blood–brain barrier); this may enable a fraction of the drug to enter the intrathecal space directly (Dale *et al* 2002a).

The nose can only accommodate volumes of 150–200 µl in each nostril, which restricts the opioid formulations suitable for intranasal administration. In addition, there is a continuous turnover/flow of mucus within the nose, which limits the time available for the drug to be absorbed (~15 min). The pharmacokinetics of relevant opioids following nasal administration have been studied in groups of healthy volunteers (Dale *et al* 2002a).

The intranasal route of administration is well established in other areas of medicine (e.g. otolaryngology). In addition, several explorative studies have looked at the use of intranasal opioids for the treatment of breakthrough pain (Zeppetella, 2000a; Pavis *et al* 2002; Fitzgibbon *et al* 2003; Kendall *et al* 2003); morphine (Pavis *et al* 2002; Fitzgibbon *et al* 2003), diamorphine (Kendall *et al* 2003), fentanyl (Zeppetella 2000a; Duncan 2002), and alfentanil (Duncan 2002) have all been reported to be useful for intranasal administration. However, methadone has been reported to be too irritant for intranasal administration (Dale *et al* 2002b). It should be noted that a commercial preparation of fentanyl citrate is currently undergoing clinical trials in Europe.

Zeppetella (2000a) reported on a small, open-label, fixed-dose study of intranasal fentanyl. The patient population consisted of 12 hospice inpatients, and the treatment regimen consisted of 20 µg fentanyl citrate (administered as 0.2 ml solution to each nostril, using two separate nasal spray bottles). Eight (67%) patients reported good or very good pain relief, and pain relief invariably occurred within

5–10 min. Moreover, nine (75%) patients reported that the pain relief with the intranasal fentanyl was greater than the pain relief with oral morphine. Two patients reported nasal discomfort/nasal itching, which subsided with ongoing usage of the spray. No patients reported any systemic opioid side effects, and none were noted by the medical staff caring for the patients.

The intranasal route is simple, does not require particularly specialized equipment, and can be used by both patients and their non-professional caregivers. Opioids can be delivered by traditional nasal spray bottles and also syringes fitted with atomizers (Figure 7.1); newer methods of delivery include devices that increase the deposition of the spray in the deeper parts of the nose, and incorporate a lock-out facility (Djupesland et al 2004). The intranasal route may be inappropriate in patients with local disease of the nose, and will be difficult to use in patients that are uncooperative.

As discussed above, one of the major problems associated with the intranasal administration of opioids is the limited availability of suitable drug formulations (i.e. concentrated solutions). Other problems relate to local side effects such as irritation (in the nose or pharynx) and taste disturbance. Little is known about the long-term effects of intranasal administration of opioids (Dale et al 2002a).

The intranasal route is only moderately attractive for the treatment of breakthrough pain for palliative care patients; Walker et al (2003) reported that 50% of patients thought that the route was acceptable for pain that was mild to moderate, whilst 68% thought that the route was acceptable for severe pain. A number of different reasons were given for not wanting to use the intranasal route (see Table 4.2).

### Fig 7.1 Atomization device (MAD™) for intranasal administration of drugs

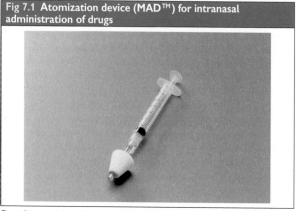

Figure 7.1 reproduced with permission from Intavent orthofix.

### 7.4.3 **Intrapulmonary administration**

The lungs have an extremely large surface area for absorption. Moreover, the alveolar surface is highly permeable, and also highly perfused with blood. (The lungs are the most highly perfused organs in the body.) All of these factors help to facilitate the absorption of drugs.

The intrapulmonary route of administration is well established in other areas of medicine (e.g. respiratory medicine, anaesthetics). Furthermore, it has been used to deliver opioids for the treatment of dyspnoea in the palliative care setting, and also to deliver opioids for the treatment of pain in the postoperative setting (Thipphawong et al 2003). However, there is little data on the use of intrapulmonary opioids for the treatment of breakthrough pain.

Zeppetella (2000b) reported on a small, case series of intrapulmonary fentanyl. The first patient was treated with 25 µg fentanyl, achieved good pain control within 15 min and did not develop any local or systemic adverse effects. The second patient was treated with 125 µg fentanyl (dose titrated), also achieved good pain control within 15 min and also did not develop any local or systemic adverse effects. In both cases, treatment was continued until either discharge (patient 2), or death (patient 1).

The intrapulmonary route is simple, does not require particularly specialized equipment and can be used by both patients and their non-professional caregivers. Opioids can be delivered by traditional nebulizers; newer methods of delivery include breath-activated delivery systems that produce small particle sizes, deliver the particles to the distal parts of the lung, and incorporate a lock-out facility (Thipphawong et al 2003). It should be noted that efficient delivery of the drug requires that the particle sizes are of the order of 1–3 µm in diameter. The intrapulmonary route may be inappropriate for certain patients, and will be difficult to use in patients that are uncooperative.

The intrapulmonary route is reasonably attractive for the treatment of breakthrough pain for palliative care patients; Walker et al (2003) reported that 60% of patients thought that the route was acceptable for pain that was mild-to-moderate in nature, whilst 75% thought that the route was acceptable for pain that was severe in nature. A number of diferent reasons were given for not wanting to use the intrapulmonary route (see Table 4.2).

## References

Dale, O., Hjortkjaer, R., Kharasch, E.D. (2002a). Nasal administration of opioids for pain management in adults. *Acta Anaesthesiologica Scandinavica*, **46**: 759–770.

Dale, O., Hoffer, C., Sheffels, P., Kharasch, E.D. (2002b). Disposition of nasal, intravenous, and oral methadone in healthy volunteers. *Clinical Pharmacology and Therapeutics*, **72**: 536–545.

Dale, O., Sheffels, P., Kharasch, E.D. (2004). Bioavailabilities of rectal and oral methadone in healthy subjects. *British Journal of Clinical Pharmacology*, **58**: 156–162.

Djupesland, P.G., Skretting, A., Windren, M., Holand, T.S. (2004). Bi-directional nasal delivery of aerosols can prevent lung deposition. *Journal of Aerosol Medicine*, **17**: 249–259.

Duncan, A. (2002). The use of fentanyl and alfentanil sprays for episodic pain. *Palliative Medicine*, **16**: 550.

Enting, R.H., Mucchiano, C., Oldenmenger, W.H., *et al.* (2005). The "pain pen" for breakthrough cancer pain: a promising treatment. *Journal of Pain and Symptom Management*, **29**: 213–217.

Fitzgibbon, D., Morgan, D., Dockter, D., *et al.* (2003). Initial pharmacokinetic, safety and efficacy evaluation of nasal morphine gluconate for breakthrough pain in cancer patients. *Pain*, **106**: 309–315.

Hanks, G., Roberts, C.J., Davies, A.N. Principles of drug use in palliative medicine. In Doyle, D., Hanks, G., Cherny, N., Calman, K., ed. *Oxford Textbook of Palliative Medicine*, (3rd edn) Oxford University Press, Oxford, 213–225.

Kendall, C.E., Davies, A.N., Forbes, K. (2003). Nasal diamorphine for 'breakthrough pain' in palliative care – a promising approach to a difficult problem [Abstract 509]. In *Proceedings of 8th Congress of the European Association for Palliative Care*. 2–5th April, Hague, Netherlands, 92.

Mercadante S, Fulfaro F. (1999). Alternatives to oral opioids for cancer pain. *Oncology* (Huntington), **13**: 215–225.

Mercadante, S., Radbruch, L., Caraceni, A., *et al.* (2002). Episodic (breakthrough) pain. Consensus Conference of an Expert Working Group of the European Association for Palliative Care. *Cancer*, **94**: 832–839.

Mercadante, S., Villari, P., Ferrera, P., *et al.* (2004). Safety and effectiveness of intravenous morphine for episodic (breakthrough) pain using a fixed ratio with the oral daily morphine dose. *Journal of Pain and Symptom Management*, **27**: 352–359.

Pavis, H., Wilcock, A., Edgecombe, J., *et al.* (2002). Pilot study of nasal morphine-chitosan for the relief of breakthrough pain in patients with cancer. *Journal of Pain and Symptom Management*, **24**: 598–602.

Sinatra, R. (2005). The fentanyl HCl patient-controlled transdermal system (PCTS): an alternative to intravenous patient-controlled analgesia in the postoperative setting. *Clinical Pharmacokinetics*, 44 (Suppl 1): 1–6.

Stevens, R.A., Ghazi, S.M. (2000). Routes of opioid analgesic therapy in the management of cancer pain. *Cancer Control*, **7**: 132–141.

Stuart-Harris, R., Joel, S.P., McDonald, P., *et al.* (2000). The pharmaco kinetics of morphine and morphine glucuronide metabolites after subcutaneous bolus injection and subcutaneous infusion of morphine. *British Journal of Clinical Pharmacology*, **49**: 207–214.

Swanson, G., Smith, J., Bulich, R., et al. (1989). Patient-controlled analgesia for chronic cancer pain in the ambulatory setting: a report of 117 patients. *Journal of Clinical Oncology*, **7**: 1903–1908.

Thipphawong, J.B., Babul, N., Morishige, R.J., et al. (2003). Analgesic efficacy of inhaled morphine in patients after bunionectomy surgery. *Anesthesiology*, **99**: 693–700.

van Hoogdalem, E., de Boer, A.G., Breimer, D.D. (1991). Pharmacokinetics of rectal drug administration, Part I. General considerations and clinical applications of centrally acting drugs. *Clinical Pharmacokinetics*, **21**: 11–26.

Viscusi, E.R., Reynolds, L., Chung, F., et al. (2004). Patient-controlled transdermal fentanyl hydrochloride vs intravenous morphine pump for postoperative pain: a randomized controlled trial. *Journal of American Medical Association*, **291**: 1333–1341.

Wagner, J.C., Souders, G.D., Coffman, L.K., Horvath, J.L. (1989). Management of chronic cancer pain using a computerized ambulatory patient-controlled analgesia pump. *Hospital Pharmacy*, **24**: 639–644.

Walker, G., Wilcock, A., Manderson, C., et al. (2003). The acceptability of different routes of administration of analgesia for breakthrough pain. *Palliative Medicine*, **17**: 219–221.

Warren, D.E. (1996). Practical use of rectal medications in palliative care. *Journal of Pain and Symptom Management*, **11**: 378–387.

Zeppetella, G. (2000a). An assessment of the safety, efficacy, and acceptability of intranasal fentanyl citrate in the management of cancer-related breakthrough pain: a pilot study. *Journal of Pain and Symptom Management*, **20**: 253–258.

Zeppetella, G. (2000b). Nebulized and intranasal fentanyl in the management of cancer-related breakthrough pain. *Palliative Medicine*, **14**: 57–58.

# Chapter 8

# Non-opioid drugs

Craig Gannon & Andrew Davies

## 8.1 Introduction

Breakthrough pains have diverse characteristics as they span all pain phenomena. This inherent diversity means that the management of breakthrough pain can effectively involve every class of drug used in analgesia. In most cases, the relevant drugs are analgesics in their own right, although their analgesic activity may not be their primary function (so-called adjuvant analgesics) (Lussier & Portenoy 2004). In other cases, the relevant drugs may not be analgesics at all, and their analgesic activity is an indirect result of their primary function, e.g. antibiotics may reduce pain by treating underlying sepsis (Bruera & MacDonald 1986).

This chapter will focus on prescribed non-opioid drugs that are commonly used in the management of cancer-related pain. The first part of the chapter will examine the evidence for non-opioid drugs in the management of relevant pain syndromes (i.e. neuropathic pain, bone pain), whilst the second part of the chapter will examine the evidence for the use of specific non-opioid drugs in the treatment of breakthrough pain episodes (e.g. midazolam, nitrous oxide). The reader is directed to more comprehensive textbooks for further information about non-opioid drugs used in the management of cancer-related pain (Doyle et al 2004; McMahon & Koltzenburg 2005).

## 8.2 Role of non-opioid drugs

Non-opioids may improve pain by a variety of different mechanisms:

- Acting as independent analgesics – non-opioid analgesics are crucial for treating opioid poorly-responsive pain.
- Supplementing opioid analgesic usage – non-opioid drugs can be used as an opioid-sparing manoeuvre, thereby avoiding the need to increase the opioid dose, and possibly allowing a decrease in the opioid dose.

- Facilitating opioid analgesic usage – non-opioid drugs can be used to combat opioid side effects, thereby avoiding the need to decrease the opioid dose, and possibly even allowing an increase in the opioid dose (e.g. psychostimulants for sedation).

In addition, non-opioid drugs may be utilized in a variety of different ways:

- 'Around the clock'/'background' analgesia – the drugs are given regularly, and their role is to treat the underlying pathological process, and so to reduce the frequency/severity of breakthrough pain episodes.
- 'Supplemental'/'breakthrough' analgesia – the drugs are given as needed, and two distinct scenarios are applicable:
  1. 'Rescue' analgesia – the drugs are given once the breakthrough pain has started, and their role is to minimize the breakthrough pain episode (i.e. spontaneous pain episodes, non-volitional incident pain episodes).
  2. 'Anticipatory' analgesia – the drugs are given in advance of the precipitating event for the breakthrough pain, and their role is to prevent/ameliorate the breakthrough pain episode (i.e. volitional incident pain episodes, procedural pain).

## 8.3 Non-opioid drugs for neuropathic pain

The standard treatment of neuropathic pain involves utilizing the WHO analgesic guidelines (WHO 1996). Studies suggest that while many patients with neuropathic pain respond to conventional analgesics (e.g. opioids) a significant number of patients also require the use of adjuvant analgesics and/or the use of other interventions (e.g. anaesthetic techniques) (Grond et al 1999). A range of adjuvant analgesics have been used in the treatment of neuropathic pain, including corticosteroids, antidepressants, anticonvulsants, local anaesthetics, anti-arrhythmic drugs, baclofen, clonidine, capsaicin, ketamine, magnesium sulphate, and bupropion (Lussier & Portenoy 2004). However, the most commonly used drugs are the antidepressants and the anticonvulsants (see below).

Making a choice from the bewildering range of options available is difficult, because of the limited data available on the effectiveness of individual drugs, and the even more limited data available on the relative effectiveness of different drugs. In practice, the choice of drug depends as much on its other characteristics (e.g. its additional effects, its adverse effects). For example, amitriptyline may be a good choice for a patient with insomnia, but it would not be a good choice for a patient with cardiac arrhythmias.

84

## 8.3.1 **Antidepressants**

### 8.3.1.1 *Tricyclic antidepressants*

The tricyclic antidepressants (TCAs) are commonly used in the management of neuropathic pain. Their analgesic effect is primarily related to the prevention of presynaptic reuptake of serotonin and noradrenaline, although other mechanisms may also be relevant (Twycross et al 2002).

There is a reasonable amount of data on the use of TCAs, and particularly on amitriptyline, in the management of neuropathic pain. Most of the data derive from studies of non-malignant pain (e.g. postherpetic neuralgia, diabetic neuropathy), but extensive clinical experience supports its use in the management of malignant pain. It should be noted that these provisos apply to many of the other adjuvant drugs used in the management of neuropathic pain (e.g. anticonvulsants).

A systematic review of the literature calculated a 'number needed to treat' (NNT) of 2 for amitriptyline (Saarto & Wiffen 2005). The NNT refers to the number of patients who need to receive a drug for one patient to achieve at least 50% relief of pain compared with placebo (Moore et al 2003). The NNT was lower for diabetic neuropathy (1.3) than for postherpetic neuralgia (2.2), but amitriptyline did not appear to be effective in human immune deficiency virus (HIV)-related neuropathy (Saarto & Wiffen 2005).

The 'number needed to harm' (NNH) for minor adverse effects was 4.6, whilst the NNH for major adverse effects (requiring withdrawal from the study) was 16 (Saarto & Wiffen 2005). The side effects of amitriptyline include drowsiness, dry mouth, blurred vision, constipation, urinary retention, heart block, and arrhythmias (Saarto & Wiffen 2005). Indeed, side effects are often the major barrier to the use of amitriptyline in the management of neuropathic pain.

Other TCAs have also been used in the management of neuropathic pain (e.g. imipramine). The data on other TCAs are much more limited, but the data that is available suggests that they may have a similar efficacy to amitriptyline (Saarto & Wiffen 2005).

### 8.3.1.2 *Selective serotonin reuptake inhibitors*

The selective serotonin reuptake inhibitors (SSRIs) have also been used in the management of neuropathic pain. Their analgesic effect is related to the prevention of presynaptic reuptake of serotonin (Twycross et al 2002).

The data on SSRIs in the management of neuropathic pain are currently relatively limited (c.f. TCAs). However, on the basis of these data, the aforementioned systematic review concluded that 'for patients who get relief from tricyclics but find the adverse effects a problem ... a trial of SSRIs ... may yield benefit' (Saarto & Wiffen 2005). It should be noted that the SSRIs are not without their side effects: problems include nausea, vomiting, dyspepsia, abdominal pain, constipation, anorexia, weight loss, and hypersensitivity reactions (Anonymous 2005). However, major side effects requiring discontinuation of treatment are relatively uncommon (Saarto & Wiffen 2005).

### 8.3.1.3 Other antidepressant drugs

Other antidepressant drugs have also been used in the management of neuropathic pain, including venlafaxine (a serotonin and noradrenaline reuptake inhibitor), and mirtazapine (a presynaptic $\alpha_2$-antagonist that increases central noradrenergic and serotonergic transmission) (Twycross et al 2002).

The data on these drugs in the management of neuropathic pain are currently very limited (c.f. TCAs, SSRIs) (Saarto & Wiffen 2005).

## 8.3.2 **Anticonvulsants**

A variety of different drugs have been used to treat epilepsy, and many of them have also been used to treat neuropathic pain. However, there is relatively little evidence to support the use of anticonvulsants in the management of neuropathic pain (c.f. antidepressants). Indeed, a systematic review of the literature concluded that 'other than trigeminal neuralgia, anticonvulsants should be withheld until other interventions have been tried' (Wiffen et al 2005a).

### 8.3.2.1 Carbamazepine

A systematic review of the use of carbamazepine in the management of neuropathic pain calculated a NNT of 1.8 for trigeminal neuralgia, but was unable to calculate a NNT for other conditions because of lack of suitable data (Wiffen et al 2005c). The NNH for minor harm was 3.7, whilst for major harm it was not statistically different from that of placebo (Wiffen et al 2005c). The side effects of carbamazepine include nausea, vomiting, dizziness, drowsiness, headache, ataxia, confusion, agitation, and visual disturbances (e.g. double vision) (Anonymous 2005).

### 8.3.2.2 Gabapentin

A further (related) systematic review of the use of gabapentin in the management of neuropathic pain calculated a combined NNT of 4.3 (Wiffen et al 2005b). (The NNT was 2.9 for diabetic neuropathy, and 3.9 for postherpetic neuralgia). The NNH for minor harm was 3.7, whilst for major harm it was not statistically different from that of placebo (Wiffen et al 2005b). The side effects of gabapentin include diarrhoea, dry mouth, dyspepsia, nausea, and vomiting (Anonymous 2005).

### 8.3.2.3 Other drugs

Other drugs that are commonly used to treat neuropathic pain include sodium valproate (limited evidence of efficacy), clonazepam (limited evidence of efficacy), and pregabalin (increasing evidence of efficacy). It should be noted that lack of evidence does not equate with lack of efficacy: clonazepam is the first-line treatment in many centres (Twycross *et al* 2002), which suggests that in day-to-day practice it as effective/well tolerated as the other neuropathic agents.

## 8.4 **Non-opioid drugs for bone pain**

The standard treatment of bone pain involves utilizing the WHO analgesic guidelines (WHO 1996). A range of adjuvant analgesics have been used in the treatment of bone pain, including corticosteroids, bisphosphonates, calcitonin, and drugs for neuropathic pain (see above) (Lussier & Portenoy 2004).

### 8.4.1 **Bisphosphonates (diphosphonates)**

Bisphosphonates are licensed for the management of osteoporosis, Paget's disease, bone metastases, and hypercalcaemia (Anonymous 2005). Bisphosphonates have a number of mechanisms of action, but their main mechanism of action relates to inhibition of osteoclast activity (leading to inhibition of bone resorption) (Twycross *et al* 2002).

A systematic review of the whole literature concluded that long-term (≥ 6 months) bisphosphonate therapy reduces skeletal morbidity associated with cancer, i.e. reduces the need for radiotherapy, reduces the incidence of fractures, and reduces the incidence of hypercalcaemia (Ross *et al* 2003). Moreover, the authors stated that bisphosphonate therapy should commence as soon as bone metastases are diagnosed and continue until 'it is no longer clinically relevant' (Ross *et al* 2003).

A subsequent systematic review of the pain literature concluded that bisphosphonate therapy provides analgesia in cancer-related bone pain (Wong & Wiffen 2002). The NNT was 11 at 4 weeks, whilst the NNT was 7 at 12 weeks. The NNH for major side effects (leading to discontinuation of treatment) was 16. The authors stated that 'there was insufficient evidence to recommend bisphosphonates for immediate effect', and 'bisphosphonates should be considered where analgesics and/or radiotherapy are inadequate for the management of painful bone metastases' (Wong & Wiffen 2002).

On the basis of the data, it would seem reasonable to prescribe bisphosphonates to patients that have already experienced morbidity as a result of bone metastases, with the primary aim of preventing further morbidity, and the secondary aim (if relevant) of treating pain. It should be noted that there are a variety of guidelines available on the use of bisphosphonates in cancer.

## 8.5 **Non-opioid drugs for breakthrough pain**

### 8.5.1 **Paracetamol (acetaminophen)**

Paracetamol is licensed for the treatment of mild to moderate pain (Anonymous 2005). Its analgesic action appears to be related to inhibition of prostaglandin production in the central nervous system (rather than in the periphery) (Twycross et al 2002).

Paracetamol is generally used as around-the-clock medication, although it may be also be used as supplemental medication. Paracetamol is recommended in the WHO pain guidelines (WHO 1996); it can be used in isolation at step 1, or in combination with opioids at step 2/3, of the WHO analgesic ladder (WHO 1996).

The evidence for the use of paracetamol in the management of cancer pain is somewhat limited (McNicol et al 2005). Stockler et al (2004) reported an additive effect when paracetamol was added to a regimen containing opioids for moderate to severe pain. However, Axelsson and Borup (2003) reported no effect when paracetamol was removed from a regimen containing opioids for moderate to severe pain.

Data from acute pain studies suggests a NNT of 3.8 for a single dose of paracetamol (1000 mg) (Moore et al 2003). The NNT for paracetamol is greater than that for the non-steroidal anti-inflammatory drugs (NSAIDs). Moreover, Ventafridda et al (1990) reported that cancer patients found paracetamol less effective than NSAIDs in a study of step 1 of the WHO analgesic ladder.

Paracetamol can be given via the oral, rectal, and intravenous routes of administration (Anonymous 2005). The onset of action of oral paracetamol is 15–30 min, and the duration of action is 4–6 hr (Twycross et al 2002). There are no contraindications to the use of paracetamol. Side effects are uncommon: reported side effects include rashes, thrombocytopenia, and leucopenia. Serious liver damage may follow an overdose of paracetamol, although it may be prevented by administration of acetylcysteine (Anonymous 2005).

### 8.5.2 **Non-steroidal anti-inflammatory drugs**

NSAIDs are licensed for the treatment of variety of painful conditions, including inflammatory conditions (e.g. rheumatoid arthritis), degenerative conditions (e.g. osteoarthritis), other painful conditions (e.g. dysmenorrhoea), and postoperative pain (Anonymous 2005). Their analgesic action appears to be related to inhibition of prostaglandin production both at the site of injury/disease (reducing inflammation), and also in the central nervous system (reducing central sensitization) (Twycross et al 2002).

NSAIDs inhibit prostaglandin production by inhibiting the enzyme cyclo-oxygenase (COX). COX is present in a number of different forms (Dickman & Ellershaw 2004). Conventional NSAIDs inhibit both COX-1 and COX-2, whilst the newer 'coxibs' specifically inhibit COX-2. It was thought that COX-2 was an inducible (by inflammation) enzyme, and that inhibition of COX-2 would be associated with minimal systemic adverse events. However, it is now known that COX-2 is also a constitutive enzyme and that inhibition of COX-2 is associated with significant systemic adverse events (see below).

NSAIDs are generally used as around-the-clock medication, although they may be also be used as supplemental medication. NSAIDs are recommended in the WHO pain guidelines (WHO 1996); they can be used in isolation at step 1, or in combination with opioids at step 2/3, of the analgesic ladder (WHO 1996). Indeed, NSAIDs have an established role as an opioid-sparing manoeuvre (Mercadante & Portenoy 2001).

Systematic reviews of oral NSAIDs have confirmed benefits in treating cancer pain (Eisenberg et al 1994; McNichol et al 2005). In the original systematic review, NSAIDs were found to be more effective than placebo, and there appeared to be no benefit to the combination of a NSAID and an opioid for mild-to-moderate pain (Eisenberg et al 1994). In the subsequent systematic review, NSAIDs were again found to be more effective than placebo, and there appeared to be a slight benefit to the combination of a NSAID and an opioid (McNichol et al 2005). However, the authors of this review were unable to comment on the relative efficacy of individual NSAIDs (i.e. calculate NNTs), or the relative tolerability of individual NSAIDs (i.e. calculate NNHs) (McNicol et al 2005).

Data from acute pain studies suggest NNTs of 2–3 for a single dose of the common oral NSAIDs (e.g. diclofenac, ibuprofen) (Moore et al 2003). It should be noted that the NNTs for NSAIDs are lower than the NNTs for other analgesic drugs (e.g. opioids for mild-to-moderate pain). Data from other studies suggest a combined NNT of 3.1 for topical NSAIDs (Moore et al 1998).

NSAIDs can be given via the oral, oral transmucosal, rectal, intravenous, intramuscular, subcutaneous, and transdermal routes of administration (Anonymous 2005; Twycross et al 2002). The onset of action and duration of action of certain oral NSAIDs is shown in Table 8.1. There are a number of contraindications to the use of NSAIDs, including hypersensitivity to aspirin/NSAIDs, coagulation defects, active peptic ulcer disease (all NSAIDs), previous peptic ulcer disease (conventional NSAIDs), ischaemic heart disease (coxibs), cerebrovascular disease (coxibs), peripheral arterial disease (coxibs), and moderate to severe congestive cardiac failure (coxibs) (Anonymous 2005). In addition, there are a number of relative contraindications relating to the known adverse effects of NSAIDs (see below) (Anonymous 2005).

Table 8.1 Clinical features of specific non steroidal anti-inflammatory drugs (Micromedex® database; Twycross et al 2002)

| Non steroidal anti-inflammatory drug | Onset of action (oral route) | Duration of action (oral route) | Comments |
|---|---|---|---|
| Ibuprofen | 15–25 min | 4–6 hr | Peak effect: 30–90 min<br>Long-acting preparations available |
| Diclofenac | 30 min | 8 hr | Long-acting preparations available |
| Ketorolac | 30 min | 5–6 hr | Peak effect: 3 hr<br>Onset of action iv/im route: 30 min |
| Naproxen | 30–60 min | Up to 12 hr | |
| Meloxicam | 90 min | – | Given once a day<br>Onset of action im route: 80 min |
| Celecoxib | 45–60 min | 4–8 hr<br>(Single dose) | Given once/twice a day |

Side effects are relatively common with NSAIDs. The major side effects of conventional NSAIDs are hypersensitivity reactions (e.g. bronchospasm), gastrointestinal problems (e.g. peptic ulceration), renal problems (e.g. renal failure), and cardiovascular problems (e.g. congestive cardiac failure) (Anonymous 2005). Gastrointestinal problems are a major cause of morbidity/mortality. However, gastrointestinal problems may be reduced by prescribing lower-risk NSAIDs (e.g. ibuprofen), by co-prescribing appropriate gastroprotection (e.g. proton-pump inhibitors), and addressing other risk factors (Dickman & Ellershaw 2004). The major side effects of coxibs are cardiovascular problems (e.g. ischaemic heart disease) (Anonymous 2005), although coxibs can also cause gastrointestinal problems (e.g. peptic ulceration) (Anonymous 2005). It should be noted that NSAIDs may cause a variety of other (less serious) side effects (Anonymous 2005).

### 8.5.3 **Midazolam**

Midazolam is a parenteral benzodiazepine, which is licensed for sedation, pre-medication for anaesthesia, and induction of anaesthesia (Anonymous 2005). Its mechanism of action involves binding to the $GABA_A$ receptor thereby enhancing the inhibitory effect of GABA (Twycross et al 2002).

As discussed, midazolam is licensed for sedation. It is used to sedate patients prior to investigative procedures (e.g. endoscopy) (Dundee et al 1984), and also prior to therapeutic procedures (e.g. wound dressing) (Jacox et al 1994). Indeed, its role in managing procedural pain has been endorsed in the EAPC expert consensus document on breakthrough pain (Mercadante et al 2002). Apart from its use in procedural pain, there is little evidence to support a wider role in the management of breakthrough pain. However, there has been a report of its use in the treatment of refractory incident pain secondary to bone metastases (del Rosario et al 2001), and there is the potential for its use in the management of breakthrough pain secondary to muscle spasm (Twycross et al 2002).

Midazolam is only available as a parenteral preparation in the United Kingdom. Nevertheless, the parenteral preparation may be administered via enteral routes (buccal, rectal), as well as via parenteral routes (intravenous, subcutaneous). It has a short onset of action (intravenous – 2–3 min; subcutaneous – 5–10 min), but a relatively long duration of action (~4 hr) (Twycross et al 2002). (It should be noted that the duration of the sedation is invariably longer than the duration of the pain.)

Contraindications to the use of midazolam include acute pulmonary insufficiency and severe respiratory depression (Anonymous 2005). The side effects of midazolam include confusion, ataxia, amnesia, headache, euphoria, hallucinations, fatigue, dizziness, vertigo, involuntary movements, paradoxical excitement, aggression, dysarthria, respiratory depression, and cardiorespiratory arrest (Anonymous 2005). In addition, there is the potential to develop tolerance and dependence to the drug; these problems only occur during chronic administration of the drug.

### 8.5.4 **Ketamine**

Ketamine is a parenteral anaesthetic agent, which is licensed for induction/maintenance of anaesthesia (Anonymous 2005) but which is also used for treatment of difficult-to-control pain (Twycross *et al* 2002). The analgesic effect of ketamine is thought to be related to blockade of the N-methyl D-aspartame (NMDA) receptor (and reduction of central sensitization/'wind-up'), although it may be related to a number of other actions including an effect on descending inhibitory pathways (Meller 1996).

Ketamine is employed in anaesthetic doses in the management of procedural pain (Jacox *et al* 1994). However, it is also employed in subanaesthetic doses in the management of other types of breakthrough pain (see below) (Carr *et al* 2004), and in the management of certain types of background pain (e.g. neuropathic pain) (Twycross *et al* 2002). In general, ketamine is used in combination with opioids in the management of background pain.

Carr *et al* (2004) reported a small, double-blind, randomized, controlled, crossover trial of intranasal ketamine in the management of breakthrough pain. The intranasal ketamine was found to be generally effective (and more effective than placebo); the onset of pain relief was within 10 min, the peak effect occurred at 40 min, and the duration of pain relief was at least 60 min. The intranasal ketamine was generally well tolerated; side effects included fatigue, dizziness, feeling of unreality, and change in taste.

The literature contains a number of case reports, case series, and clinical trials of the use of ketamine in the management of cancer pain. As discussed above, ketamine is generally used in combination with opioids in the management of background pain. It has been reported that ketamine can restore opioid responsiveness and prevent the development of opioid tolerance. However, a recent systematic review of the literature concluded that the evidence was 'insufficient to assess the benefits and harms of ketamine' (Bell *et al* 2003).

Ketamine has been given by the oral, intramuscular (licensed), intravenous (licensed), subcutaneous, intranasal, and spinal routes of administration. The side effects of ketamine include involuntary muscle contractions, hypertension (previous history is a relative contraindication), tachycardia, and hallucinations (previous history is a relative contraindication) (Anonymous 2005). Hallucinations can be prevented/treated with benzodiazepines (e.g. diazepam) (Anonymous 2005).

### 8.5.5 **Nitrous oxide**

Nitrous oxide is an inhalational anaesthetic, which is licensed for maintenance of anaesthesia and management of pain (at subanaesthetic doses) (Anonymous 2005). Its mechanism of action has not been completely elucidated: one hypothesis is that nitrous oxide causes the release of opioid peptides in the periaqueductal grey area of the midbrain, which leads to activation of descending noradrenergic pathways, which in turn leads to modulation of pain impulses in the dorsal horn of the spinal cord (Entonox® Reference Guide).

As discussed, nitrous oxide is licensed for the management of pain. It is used to treat patients with pain related to pathological processes (e.g. trauma) (Donen et al 1982), and also pain due to therapeutic procedures (e.g. wound dressings) (Jacox et al 1994). Apart from its use in procedural pain, there is some evidence to support a wider role in the management of breakthrough pain. Thus there is a small case series (Keating & Kundrat 1996) and a small double-blind, randomized, controlled, crossover trial (Parlow et al 2005), which support the use of nitrous oxide in the management of breakthrough pain. However, another small case series was contradictory (Enting et al 2002). Nevertheless, its role in managing incident pain has been endorsed in the EAPC expert consensus document on breakthrough pain (Mercadante et al 2002).

Nitrous oxide is co-administered with oxygen (50:50 mixture for analgesia): it comes in a portable gas cylinder with a breath-activated valve, and may be used with either a face mask or a mouth piece. It has a short onset of action (<<1 min), a quick time to peak effect (2 min), and a short duration of action (5–40 min: subjective measures–objective measures) (Entonox® Reference Guide).

Contraindications to the use of nitrous oxide include the presence of a pneumothorax: the nitrous oxide can diffuse into the pneumothorax, causing an increase in the volume/pressure of the pneumothorax (Anonymous 2005). Side effects include sedation (7.6%), dizziness (10.3%), nausea (5.7%), excitation (3.7%) and 'numbness' (0.3%) (Entonox® Reference Guide). Nitrous oxide can interfere with vitamin $B_{12}$, and chronic usage may result in megaloblastic anaemia and neurological problems (polyneuropathy, spinal cord degeneration) (Anonymous 2005; Doran et al 2004). In addition, there is the potential to develop tolerance to the drug; this problem may occur during acute administration of the drug (Ramsay et al 2005).

### 8.5.6 **Other agents**

It should be noted that a variety of other sedative/anaesthetic agents have also been used to treat procedural pain (e.g. propofol, barbiturates) (Jacox et al 1994).

# References

Anonymous (2005). *British National Formulary 50*. BMJ Publishing Group Ltd and Royal Pharmaceutical Society of Great Britain, London.

Axelsson, B., Borup S. (2003). Is there an additive analgesic effect of paracetamol at step 3? A double-blind randomized controlled study. *Palliative Medicine*, **17**: 724–725.

Bell, R., Eccleston, C., Kalso, E. (2003). Ketamine as an adjuvant to opioids for cancer pain. *Cochrane Database of Systematic Reviews (1)*, CD003351.

Bruera, E., MacDonald, N. (1986). Intractable pain in patients with advanced head and neck tumors: a possible role of local infection. *Cancer Treatment Reports*, **70**: 691–692.

Carr, D.B., Goudas, L.C., Denman, W.T. *et al.* (2004). Safety and efficacy of intranasal ketamine for the treatment of breakthrough pain in patients with chronic pain: a randomized, double-blind, placebo-controlled, crossover study. *Pain*, **108**: 17–27.

del Rosario, M.A., Martin, A.S., Ortega, J.J., Feria, M. (2001). Temporary sedation with midazolam for control of severe incident pain. *Journal of Pain and Symptom Management*, **21**: 439–442.

Dickman, A., Ellershaw, J. (2004). NSAIDs: gastroprotection or selective COX-2 inhibitor? *Palliative Medicine*, **18**: 275–286.

Donen, N., Tweed, W.A., White, D., *et al.* (1982). Pre-hospital analgesia with Entonox. *Canadian Anaesthetists' Society Journal*, **29**: 275–279.

Doran, M., Rassam, S.S., Jones, L.M., Underhill, S. (2004). Toxicity after inhalation of nitrous oxide for analgesia. *British Medical Journal*, **328**: 1364–1365.

Doyle, D., Hanks, G., Cherny, N., Calman, K. (2004). *Oxford Textbook of Palliative Medicine* (3rd edn) Oxford University Press, Oxford.

Dundee, J.W., Halliday, N.J., Harper, K.W., Brogden, R.N. (1984). Midazolam. A review of its pharmacological properties and therapeutic use. *Drugs*, **28**: 519–543.

Eisenberg, E., Berkey, C.S., Carr, D.B., *et al.* (1994). Efficacy and safety of nonsteroidal antiinflammatory drugs for cancer pain: a meta-analysis. *Journal of Clinical Oncology*, **12**: 2756–2765.

Enting, R.H., Oldenmenger, W.H., van der Rijt, C.C., *et al.* (2002). Nitrous oxide is not beneficial for breakthrough cancer pain. *Palliative Medicine*, **16**: 257–259.

Grond, S., Radbruch, L., Meuser, T., *et al* (1999). Assessment and treatment of neuropathic cancer pain. Pain, **79**: 15–20.

Jacox, A., Carr D.B., Payne, R., *et al.* (1994). *Management of Cancer Pain*. Agency for Health Care Policy and Research, Rockville.

Keating, H.J., Kundrat, M. (1996). Patient-controlled analgesia with nitrous oxide in cancer pain. *Journal of Pain and Symptom Management*, **11**: 126–130.

Lussier, D., Portenoy, R.K. (2004). Adjuvant analgesics in pain management. In Doyle D., Hanks, G., Cherny ,N., Calman, K., ed. *Oxford*

*Textbook of Palliative Medicine* (3rd edn). Oxford University Press, Oxford, 349–378.

McMahon, S., Koltzenburg, M. (2005). *Wall and Melzack's Textbook of Pain*. Churchill Livingstone, Philadelphia.

McNicol, E., Strassels, S.A., Goudas, L., *et al.* (2005). NSAIDS or paracetamol, alone or combined with opioids, for cancer pain. *Cochrane Database of Systematic Reviews*, (2), CD005180.

Meller, S.T. (1996). Ketamine: relief from chronic pain through actions at the NMDA receptor? *Pain*, **68**: 435–436.

Mercadante, S., Portenoy, R.K. (2001). Opioid poorly-responsive cancer pain. Part 3. Clinical strategies to improve opioid responsiveness. *Journal of Pain and Symptom Management*, **21**: 338–354.

Mercadante, S., Radbruch, L., Caraceni, A., *et al.* (2002). Episodic (break-through) pain. Consensus Conference of an Expert Working Group of the European Association for Palliative Care. *Cancer*, **94**: 832–839.

Moore, R.A., Tranmer, M.R., Carroll, D. *et al.* (1998). Quantitative systematic review of topically applied non-steroidal anti-inflammatory drugs. *British Medical Journal*, **316**: 333–338.

Moore, A., Edwards, J., Barden, J., McQuay, H. (2003). *Bandolier's Little Book of Pain*. Oxford University Press, Oxford.

Parlow, J.L., Milne, B., Tod, D.A., *et al.* (2005). Self-administered nitrous oxide for the management of incident pain in terminally ill patients: a blinded case series. *Palliative Medicine*, **19**: 3–8.

Ramsay D.S., Leroux, B.G., Rothen, M., *et al.* (2005). Nitrous oxide analgesia in humans: acute and chronic tolerance. *Pain*, **114**: 19–28.

Ross, J.R., Saunders, Y., Edmonds, P.M., *et al.* (2003). Systematic review of role of bisphosphonates on skeletal morbidity in metastatic cancer. *British Medical Journal*, **327**: 469–472.

Saarto, T., Wiffen P. (2005). Antidepressants for neuropathic pain. *Cochrane Database of Systematic Reviews*, (**3**): CD005454.

Stockler, M., Vardy, J. Pillai, A., Warr, D. (2004). Acetaminophen (paracetamol) improves pain and well-being in people with advanced cancer already receiving a strong opioid regimen: a randomized, double-blind, placebo-controlled, cross-over trial. *Journal of Clinical Oncology*, **22**: 3389–3394.

Twycross, R., Wilcock, A., Charlesworth, S., Dickman, A. (2002). *Palliative Care Formulary*, (2nd edn). Radcliffe Medical Press, Abingdon.

Ventafridda, V., De Conno, F., Panerai, A.E., *et al.* (1990). Non-steroidal anti-inflammatory drugs as the first step in cancer pain therapy: double-blind, within patient study comparing nine drugs. *Journal of International Medical Research*, **18**: 21–29.

World Health Organization (1996). *Cancer Pain Relief* (2nd edn). World Health Organization, Geneva.

Wiffen, P., Collins, S., McQuay, H., *et al.* (2005a). Anticonvulsant drugs for acute and chronic pain. *Cochrane Database of Systematic Reviews*, (3): CD001133.

CHAPTER 8 **Non-opioid drugs**

Wiffen, P.J., McQuay, H.J., Edwards, J.E., Moore, R.A. (2005b). Gabapentin for acute and chronic pain. *Cochrane Database of Systematic Reviews*, (3): CD005452.

Wiffen, P.J., McQuay, H.J., Moore, R.A. (2005c). Carbamazepine for acute and chronic pain. *Cochrane Database of Systematic Reviews*, (3): CD005451.

Wong, R., Wiffen, P.J. (2002). Bisphosphonates for the relief of pain secondary to bone metastases. *Cochrane Database of Systematic Reviews*, (2): CD002068.

# Chapter 9

# Other therapeutic interventions

Nicholas Christelis & Jackie Filshie

## 9.1 Introduction

A wide variety of non-pharmacological interventions have been used to treat cancer-related pain (Doyle et al 2004). This chapter will focus on anaesthetic interventions used to treat difficult pain problems associated with breakthrough pain episodes. However, this chapter will also touch on non-pharmacological interventions used to treat actual breakthrough pain episodes (e.g. transcutaneous electrical nerve stimulation: TENS).

Anaesthetic interventions are usually intended to be an adjuvant to systemic analgesic treatment. Indeed, these interventions have been suggested to be the fourth step of the WHO analgesic ladder (Miguel 2000). However, these interventions have a limited role in the management of cancer pain. For example, only 11% of patients required anaesthetic interventions to help to control their pain in a validation study of the WHO analgesic guidelines (Zech et al 1995).

## 9.2 General principles

The usual indications for these anaesthetic techniques include pain that is poorly responsive to systemic analgesics, or the development of intolerable side effects caused by them. Thus, anaesthetic techniques may allow patients to experience better pain relief from current drug doses, or may allow patients to reduce drug doses thereby reducing drug side effects. A patient with a short life expectancy, and with limited time available for the safe titration of systemic analgesics, may also be considered for these anaesthetic techniques (Hicks & Simpson 2004). Nerve blockade may be useful in patients with localized pain, or pain with a neuropathic element that is not responding to adjuvant analgesics. Neuraxial analgesic delivery may be useful in patients with pain from locally aggressive tumours in the abdomen and pelvis, or in patients with pain from pathological fractures that are not suitable for surgical fixation.

Before complex anaesthetic interventions such as neuraxial analgesia delivery are considered, available alternatives such as disease-modifying treatments should be considered. Furthermore, when anaesthetic interventions are considered, the simplest method should be considered first. For example, stimulation-based analgesic techniques (TENS, acupuncture) might precede nerve blockade.

As with any form of treatment, appropriate patient selection is necessary. The assessment process involves taking a history, performing an examination, and the utilization of relevant investigations. The history should include a detailed assessment of the pain, and the examination should include a full neurological assessment (Bruera & Neumann 2003). Laboratory investigations will include a platelet count and a coagulation screen to identify potential bleeding problems. Radiological investigations may include computerized tomography (CT) scanning or magnetic resonance imaging (MRI): these tests are necessary to identify anatomical distortion and other potential problems relating to the chosen anaesthetic technique (Erdine 2005).

Absolute contraindications to anaesthetic interventions include patient refusal, non-correctable coagulopathy, and localized infection at the proposed site of needle entry.

The use of complex anaesthetic interventions such as neuraxial analgesia delivery requires a coordinated approach from a multidisciplinary pain management team, which will usually comprise specialist consultants (pain management, palliative care), nurses, physiotherapists, and psychologists. Appropriate facilities and resources to apply these techniques are necessary. These include laboratory and radiology services. Also required are appropriate resources to monitor and follow up patients who have received these interventions. These patients require a coordinated support system that allows easy access to the hospital multidisciplinary team and to other healthcare professionals, such as general practitioners and district nurses in the community.

## 9.3 **Peripheral nerve blockade**

Local anaesthetic peripheral nerve blockades are probably the most common interventions used in cancer pain management. Examples of useful techniques include intercostal nerve blockade for rib pain, suprascapular nerve blockade for shoulder pain, brachial plexus blockade for upper extremity pain, and sciatic/femoral nerve blockade for lower extremity pain. They are relatively easy to perform, and carry a low incidence of serious side effects.

Local anaesthetic nerve blockade can produce anaesthesia/analgesia lasting up to 12 hours, although it has been observed that the analgesic effect may sometimes outlast the anaesthetic effect by days or weeks (Boys *et al* 1993). Corticosteroids may be combined with local anaesthetics with the aim of providing additional/longer-lasting analgesia (Twycross 1994). A modification of the 'single-shot' technique involves the placement of a catheter for the administration of repeated boluses, or continuous infusion, of local anaesthetic (Aguilar *et al* 1995; Fischer *et al* 1996).

In order to provide more prolonged analgesia, a temporary block using local anaesthetic may be followed up by a more permanent block using a neurolytic agent. Neurolytic agents include alcohol (3–100%), phenol (5–15%) and glycerol. Neurolytic agents damage the nerves in different ways, but all have the potential to be reversible, thereby causing the pain to return after a period of time (~3–4 months) (Williams 2003).

One complication of neurolytic blockade is the development of post neurolysis deafferentation neuralgia (neuropathic pain), which may be permanent. When life expectancy is more than a few months, non-chemical neurolytic blockade (e.g. radiofrequency ablation, cryoablation) is preferable to chemical neurolytic blockade (e.g. alcohol, phenol), as the incidence of neuropathic pain has been found to be reduced with these techniques (Erdine 2005, Goh 2005).

It should be noted that a successful local anaesthetic block does not guarantee a successful neurolytic block, since there is no guarantee that the neurolytic agent will be placed at precisely the same location as the local anaesthetic, or that the neurolytic agent will behave in the same manner as the local anaesthetic.

## 9.4 **Neuraxial analgesia delivery**

The epidural and intrathecal (subarachnoid) routes are the two main methods used to deliver neuraxial blockade (Erdine 2005). The epidural route remains the preferred route for neuraxial analgesia delivery in cancer pain (Baker *et al* 2004). However, there is growing evidence that opioids delivered by the intrathecal route may provide better analgesia, and may be safer, than opioids delivered by the epidural route (Dahm *et al* 1998; Gestin *et al* 1997). As a result, use of the intrathecal route is increasingly, and it is even being used exclusively in some units (Baker *et al* 2004).

The epidural route should probably be avoided in patients with known epidural disease, since this may interfere with the positioning of the catheter, and also with the free flow of the analgesic agents. In addition, the epidural route may not be suitable for long-term use because of the potential for development of local fibrosis, which may also interfere with the flow of the analgesic agents (Wagemans et al 1997). Epidural opioids need to be given in higher dosage than intrathecal opioids and, consequently, epidural opioid delivery may be associated with greater side effects compared with intrathecal opioid delivery.

Drug delivery is via a percutaneous catheter and external pump or via a totally implantable drug delivery system. Percutaneous catheters may be tunneled under the skin (to exit at a distant site): tunneled catheters are more robust and have a lower incidence of infection than non-tunneled catheters (Arbit & Pannullo 2003). Implantable delivery systems are reserved for longer-term intrathecal therapy in those with a prolonged life expectancy. Implantable delivery systems have a high initial cost, but appear to be cost-effective in the long term (several months to years) (Swarm et al 2004).

Neuraxial analgesia is best established by a constant infusion (Baker et al 2004) as adverse events frequently relate to bolus delivery of the analgesic agents, particularly when treatment is first instituted. Large boluses have caused cardiorespiratory arrest (Piquet et al 1998). The newer external pumps, and some implantable delivery systems, offer the ability to deliver low-dose, patient-controlled boluses of the analgesic agents, which may provide improved analgesia with less systemic side effects.

Neuraxial analgesia is usually commenced with opioid analgesics. A variety of opioids have been used for neuraxial analgesia although morphine has been the traditional opioid of choice (Hicks & Simpson 2004). Morphine is relatively hydrophilic, which results in a relatively slower onset of action (epidural route), longer duration of action, and greater relative potency compared with other opioids (Hicks & Simpson 2004). Morphine is also more likely to spread in a cranial direction, which may extend the level of analgesia, but also increase the risk of respiratory depression. Other opioids that have been used in this setting, include fentanyl, sufentanil, hydromorphone, oxycodone, and methadone.

Neuraxial delivery of opioids produces inadequate analgesia in 10–30% of patients (Malone 1985). In these cases, the co-administration of a local anaesthetic may provide additional analgesia (Du Pen et al 1992). Indeed, there is now a growing trend to use combination treatment from the outset. Local anaesthetics and opioids may act synergistically, allowing lower doses of the individual drugs to be used, which may limit the side effects of the individual drugs (Yaksh & Mulberg, 1994).

It should be noted that low-dose infusions of local anaesthetics (e.g. bupivacaine, ropivacaine) can provide adequate analgesia without producing significant sensory disturbance, or motor impairment (Dahm et al 2000). However, boluses of local anaesthetics can produce unpleasant paraesthesia and symptomatic hypotension.

Other analgesic agents may also be delivered via the neuraxial route, including clonidine, baclofen, midazolam, ketamine, and ziconotide (Swarm et al 2004). Clonidine, an alpha 2 adrenoreceptor agonist, is a useful adjunct to spinal opioids, particularly in patients with neuropathic pain (Eisenach et al 1995).

The early complications of these techniques include catheter misplacement, cerebrospinal fluid (CSF) leak, bleeding, and infection. The later complications include catheter kinking, catheter displacement, or catheter obstruction by fibrosis (epidural catheters) or granuloma formation (intrathecal catheters). Rarely, spinal cord compression is caused by haematomas, abscesses, or granulomas (Cabbell et al 1998). Other complications relate to the analgesic agents employed. Long-term intrathecal opioid infusion can lead to tolerance or hyperalgesia (Osenbach & Harvey 2001).

## 9.5 **Neuromodulation**

### 9.5.1 **Transcutaneous electrical nerve stimulation**

TENS is a potent form of nerve stimulation (Thompson 1998). It acts by inhibiting transmission of pain impulses from the periphery to the central nervous system by stimulating peripheral sensory nerve fibres (Bercovitch & Waller 2004). Other mechanisms may also be relevant, including activation of descending inhibitory pathways and activation of the sympathetic nervous system.

A basic TENS machine consists of a small, battery-operated, electrical pulse generator and a set of electrodes (Figure 9.1) (Bercovitch & Waller 2004). Most machines have the ability to vary the intensity, frequency, pulse duration, and type of output (i.e. continuous pulses, bursts of pulses, modulation/variation of pulses). The optimal settings to obtain pain relief vary from patient to patient, and need to be determined by trial and error in each patient (Thompson, 1998).

TENS is a well-established treatment for cancer pain. However, there is relatively little evidence to support its use in the treatment of cancer pain (Bercovitch & Waller 2004). TENS has been used to treat background pain and episodes of breakthrough pain (Filshie & Thompson 2000; Zeppetella & Ribeiro 2003). TENS is not used as often as perhaps it might, partly because of the time and effort needed to find the optimal electrode placement/generator settings (Thompson 1998).

TENS can be used to treat any localized pain of somatic or neuropathic origin, providing paraesthesia can be generated in the region of the pain, or within the same or a closely-related dermatome (Woolf & Thompson 1994). It can be difficult to predict the response to TENS; a therapeutic trial is the only way to determine if TENS will be successful or not ( Johnson et al 1991).

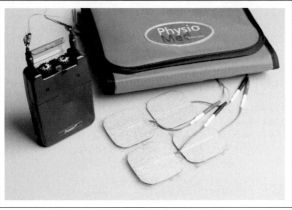

**Fig 9.1 Physio-Med TPN 200 PP TENS machine**

Contraindications to TENS include skin inflammation, skin infection and the presence of a cardiac pacemaker (Bercovitch & Waller 2004). TENS should not be used over the anterior neck as stimulation of the laryngeal nerves may lead to laryngospasm, whilst stimulation of the carotid sinus may lead to hypotension. Serious complications are rare. Adverse effects include skin irritation, skin burns, and allergy (to electrode gel/tape) (Bercovitch & Waller 2004).

### 9.5.2 Spinal cord stimulation

The analgesic mechanism of spinal cord stimulation is not fully understood, but is thought to work by activating endogenous inhibitory systems within the central nervous system (Swarm et al 2004).

Spinal cord stimulation involves implanting electrodes in the epidural space at the spinal level corresponding to the site of pain. Nowadays, electrode placement is performed percutaneously in an awake patient, in order to ensure optimal electrode placement (Stannard 2003). Initially, a trial of spinal cord stimulation is undertaken using a temporary external system. If this proves successful, the temporary external system can then be replaced by a fully implantable system.

Although numerous studies document the efficacy of spinal cord stimulation, there are few data on the use of spinal cord stimulation for cancer pain. One series concluded that spinal cord stimulation was not useful for cancer pain (Meglio et al 1989), but the results were equivocal in an earlier series (Krainick & Thouden 1974).

The main complications of spinal cord stimulation are infection (<1%) and technical failures, such as migration of electrodes and breakage of electrodes.

## 9.6 Neuroablation

Neuroablation (neurolytic blockade) is defined as the physical interruption or destruction of neurones and pathways conducting pain impulses. It can be performed chemically, thermally, or surgically.

Over the past two decades the role of neurolytic blockade has diminished, as neuraxial analgesic delivery has become more established. Nevertheless, there remains a limited role for neurolytic blockade in patients with localized intractable pain, and with a relatively short life expectancy (Goh 2005).

### 9.6.1 Peripheral neurolytic blockade
See above.

### 9.6.2 Neurolytic blockade of sympathetic nervous system
The sympathetic nervous system plays a role in the modulation of certain pain impulses (Swarm et al 2004). Moreover, the sympathetic chain and ganglia are traversed by visceral nociceptive fibres. Hence, blockade of the sympathetic nervous system may be useful in certain types of pain, such as visceral or neuropathic pain.

It has recently been suggested that neurolytic sympathetic blockade (of coeliac plexus, lumbar plexus, or superior hypogastric plexus) be considered earlier, rather than later, in the management of abdominal or pelvic cancer (de Oliveira et al 2004). A diagnostic block using a local anaesthetic is sometimes used to establish the relative contribution of the sympathetic system to the aetiology of the pain.

#### 9.6.2.1 Coeliac plexus blockade
Coeliac plexus blockade is probably the most established of all the neurolytic pain blockades. It can be useful for visceral pain arising from the pancreas and other upper abdominal structures (Swarm et al 2004).

Needle placement is performed using radiographic imaging such as fluoroscopy or CT in sedated or anaesthetized patients. Endoscopic ultrasound (EUS) guided neurolytic coeliac plexus blockade has recently been described (Arcidiacono & Rossi 2004).

A meta-analysis of relevant studies found that 89% of patients had 'good to excellent' pain relief during the first 2 weeks post blockade, that ~90% of patients had 'partial to complete' pain relief at 3 months post blockade, and that 70–90% of patients had 'partial to complete' pain relief up until death (Eisenberg et al 1995).

Certain adverse effects are common after coeliac plexus block: these include orthostatic hypotension (63%) and diarrhoea (44%)

(Swarm *et al* 2004). These effects are usually transient, and generally mild in nature, requiring little or no treatment. Other more serious, although uncommon, complications have also been reported. These include paraplegia (<1%), aortic dissection, generalized seizures and circulatory arrest (Davies 1993; Kaplan *et al* 1995).

#### 9.6.2.2 *Lumbar sympathetic blockade*

Lumbar sympathetic blockade can be useful for neuropathic pain arising from the lower extremities, and also visceral pain arising from lower abdominal and pelvic structures (Brevik *et al* 1998).

#### 9.6.2.3 *Superior hypogastric blockade*

This type of blockade may be useful in patients with visceral pain from pelvic structures (Swarm *et al* 2004).

#### 9.6.2.4 *Ganglion impar (ganglion of Walther) blockade*

This type of blockade may be useful in patients with perineal pain, and rectal pain (Swarm *et al* 2004).

### 9.6.3 **Neurolytic blockade of the central nervous system**

#### 9.6.3.1 *Intrathecal (subarachnoid) neurolysis*

The aim of intrathecal neurolysis is to disrupt the anterolateral spinothalamic tracts. These blocks can be effective for bilateral perineal pain ('saddle pain'), and also for unilateral torso pain (Patt & Cousins 1998).

#### 9.6.3.2 *Cervical cordotomy*

The aim of cervical cordotomy is to disrupt the spinothalamic tracts just below the medulla oblongata. It is particularly helpful for unilateral pain from a mesothelioma (Kanpolat *et al* 2002), or a Pancoast's tumour (Ischia *et al* 1985) that have failed to respond to other treatment. It may also be helpful for other unilateral pains involving the chest, upper extremity, pelvis, and lower extremity (Hassenbach & Cherny 2004).

A variety of other neurolytic procedures have been reported, although many of them are now rarely used (Hassenbach & Cherny 2004; Swarm *et al* 2004).

## 9.7 **Other interventions**

### 9.7.1 **Acupuncture**

Acupuncture is a form of sensory stimulation, which relies on Aδ nerve stimulation using percutaneous needles to produce analgesia via neuromodulation of pain pathways and numerous endogenous spinal and supraspinal analgesic mechanisms (Filshie & Thompson 2004).

Acupuncture has been shown to raise the pain threshold (Brockhaus & Elger 1990), as well as reduce experimentally induced pain (White 1999) and acute pain (Kotani et al 2001). It is regularly used to treat cancer pain, although there is a lack of good evidence to support its role in the treatment of cancer pain (Filshie & Thompson 2004). One of the main reasons for the lack of evidence is the difficulty of undertaking controlled/blinded trials of acupuncture (Filshie & Thompson 2004).

Acupuncture can provide acute pain relief, as well as more prolonged pain relief (i.e. days to weeks) (Filshie & Thompson 2004). Indeed, it may be more helpful in treating the underlying pain state than in treating actual breakthrough pain episodes. Acupuncture is especially useful for pain of musculoskeletal origin (Baldry 2004).

A variety of techniques may be utilized, involving different acupuncture points, different modes of stimulation (e.g. minimal stimulation, vigorous stimulation), different durations of stimulation, and variable course lengths (Filshie & Thompson 2004). A typical course of acupuncture will involve weekly treatments for 6 weeks, followed by 'top-up' treatments every few weeks (Filshie & Thompson 2004).

Contraindications to acupuncture have been described in cancer patients, and include thrombocytopenia, neutropenia, lymphoedema, local infection, and local tumour (Filshie 2001). Furthermore, needling should not be performed near an unstable spine, since any muscle relaxation may worsen the spinal stability. Acupuncture has been shown to be safe in a number of large prospective studies with the most common adverse effects being post treatment pain (~1%), bleeding/bruising (~3%), and somnolence (MacPherson et al 2001; White et al 2001).

### 9.7.2 Miscellaneous interventions for bone pain

A variety of other interventional techniques have been reported to be useful in treating pain secondary to localised bone disease, although most of them have not been subjected to rigorous scientific investigation These include: • Corticosteroid instillation (Rousseff & Simeonov 2004) • Alcohol instillation (Gangi et al 1996) • Phenol instillation (Gangi et al 1996) • Cryoablation (Callstrom et al 2006) • Radiofrequency ablation (Goetz et al 2004) • Laser ablation (Callstrom et al 2006) • Cementoplasty/vertebroplasty (Gangi et al 2003) – this technique involves injecting methylmethacrylate cement into the affected bone • Balloon kyphoplasty (Fourney et al 2003) – this technique is similar to vertebroplasty but involves initially inflating a balloon within the affected bone (to improve the alignment of the bone and also to create a cavity for the cement within the bone).

### 9.7.3 Miscellaneous interventions for breakthrough pain episodes

A variety of other non-pharmacological methods have also been reported useful in treating breakthrough pain episodes although, again, most of them have not been subjected to rigorous scientific investigation: • Rubbing/massage (Fine & Busch 1998; Swanwick *et al* 2001) • Application of heat (Fine & Busch 1998; Swanwick *et al* 2001) • Application of cold (Fine & Busch 1998; Petzke *et al* 1999) • Distraction techniques (Petzke *et al* 1999; Portenoy 1997) • Relaxation techniques (Fine & Busch 1998; Portenoy 1997) • Hypnotherapy/hypnosis (Liossi 2000; Wild & Espie 2004).

The non-invasive nature of these interventions means that it is always worth a therapeutic trial of these interventions. Furthermore, patients find these types of treatment highly acceptable for managing their breakthrough pain, particularly as they have often used them for managing other types of pain (e.g. benign musculoskeletal pain).

# References

Aguilar, J.L., Domingo, V., Samper, D., *et al*. (1995). Long-term brachial plexus anesthesia using a subcutaneous implantable injection system. Case report. *Regional Anesthesia*, **20**: 242–245.

Arbit, E., Pannullo, S. (2003). In Sykes, N., Fallon, M.T., Patt, R.B., ed. *Clinical Pain Management. Cancer Pain*, Oxford University Press, New York, 259–267.

Arcidiacono, P.G., Rossi, M. (2004). Celiac plexus neurolysis. *Journal of the Pancreas*, **5**: 315–321.

Baker, L., Lee, M., Regnard, C. *et al*. (2004). Evolving spinal analgesia practice in palliative care. *Palliative Medicine*, **18**: 507–515.

Baldry, P.E. (2004). *Acupuncture, Trigger Points and Musculoskeletal Pain* (3rd edn) Churchill Livingstone, Edinburgh.

Bercovitch, M., Waller, A. (2004). Transcutaneous electrical nerve stimulation (TENS). In Doyle, D., Hanks, G., Cherny, N., Calman, K., ed. *Oxford Textbook of Palliative Medicine* (3rd edn) Oxford University Press, Oxford, 405–410.

Boys, L., Peat, S.J., Hanna, M.H., Burn, K. (1993). Audit of neural blockade for palliative care patients in an acute unit. *Palliative Medicine*, **7**: 205–211.

Breivik, H., Cousins, M.J., Lofstrom, B.J. (1998). Sympathetic neural blockade of upper and lower extremity. In Cousins, M.J., Bridenbaugh, P.O., ed. *Neural Blockade in Clinical Anaesthesia and Management of Pain* (3rd edn) Lippincott-Raven, Philadelphia, 411–445.

Brockhaus, A., Elger, C.E. (1990). Hypalgesic efficacy of acupuncture on experimental pain in man. Comparison of laser acupuncture and needle acupuncture. *Pain*, **43**: 181–185.

Bruera, E., Neumann, C.M. (2003). In Sykes, N., Fallon, M.T., Patt, R.B., ed. *Clinical Pain Management. Cancer Pain* Oxford University Press, New York, 63–71.

Cabbell, K.L., Taren, J.A., Sagher, O. (1998). Spinal cord compression by catheter granulomas in high-dose intrathecal morphine therapy: case report. *Neurosurgery*, **42**: 1176–1180.

Callstrom, M.R., Charboneau, J.W., Goetz, M.P., et al. (2006). Image-guided ablation of painful metastatic bone tumors: a new and effective approach to a difficult problem. *Skeletal Radiology*, **35**: 1–15.

Dahm, P., Nitescu, P., Appelgren, L., Curelaru, I. (1998). Efficacy and technical complications of long-term continuous intraspinal infusions of opioid and/or bupivacaine in refractory nonmalignant pain: a comparison between the epidural and the intrathecal approach with externalized or implanted catheters and infusion pumps. *Clinical Journal of Pain*, 14: 4–16.

Dahm, P., Lundborg, C., Janson, M. et al. (2000). Comparison of 0.5% intrathecal bupivacaine with 0.5% intrathecal ropivacaine in the treatment of refractory cancer and noncancer pain conditions: results from a prospective, crossover, double-blind, randomized study. *Regional Anesthesia and Pain Medicine*, **25**: 480–487.

Davies, D.D. (1993). Incidence of major complications of neurolytic coeliac plexus block. *Journal of the Royal Society of Medicine*, **86**: 264–266.

de Oliveira, R., dos Reis, M.P., Prado, W.A. (2004). The effects of early or late neurolytic sympathetic plexus block on the management of abdominal or pelvic cancer pain. *Pain*, **110**: 400–408.

Doyle, D., Hanks, G., Cherny, N., Calman, K. (2004). *Oxford Textbook of Palliative Medicine* (3rd edn) Oxford University Press, Oxford.

Du Pen, S.L., Karasch, E.D., Williams, A., et al. (1992). Chronic epidural bupivacaine-opioid infusion in intractable cancer pain. Pain, **49**: 293–300.

Eisenach, J.C., DuPen, S., Dubois, M., et al (1995). Epidural clonidine analgesia for intractable cancer pain. The Epidural Clonidine Study Group. *Pain*, **61**: 391–399.

Eisenberg, E., Carr, D.B., Chalmers, T.C. (1995). Neurolytic celiac plexus block for treatment of cancer pain: a meta-analysis. *Anesthesia and Analgesia*, **80**: 290–295.

Erdine, S. (2005). Interventional treatment of cancer pain. *European Journal of Cancer Supplements*, **3**: 97–106.

Filshie, J. (2001). Safety aspects of acupuncture in palliative care. *Acupuncture in Medicine*, **19**: 117–122.

Filshie, J., Thompson, J.W. (2000). Acupuncture and TENS. In Simpson, K.H., Budd, K., ed. *Cancer Pain Management. A Comprehensive Approach*. Oxford University Press, Oxford, 188–223.

Filshie, J., Thompson, J.W. (2004). Acupuncture. In Doyle, D., Hanks, G., Cherny, N., Calman, K., ed. *Oxford Textbook of Palliative Medicine* (3rd edn). Oxford University Press, Oxford, 410–424.

Fine, P.G., Busch, M.A. (1998). Characterization of breakthrough pain by hospice patients and their caregivers. *Journal of Pain and Symptom Management*, **16**: 179–183.

Fischer, H.B., Peters, T.M., Fleming, I.M., Else, T.A. (1996). Peripheral nerve catheterization in the management of terminal cancer pain. *Regional Anesthesia*, **21**: 482–485.

Fourney, D.R., Schomer, D.F., Nader, R., et al. (2003). Percutaneous vertebroplasty and kyphoplasty for painful vertebral body fractures in cancer patients. *Journal of Neurosurgery*, **98** (1 Suppl): 21–30.

Gangi, A., Dietemann, J.L., Schultz, A., et al. (1996). Interventional radiologic procedures with CT guidance in cancer pain management. *Radiographics*, **16**: 1289–1304.

Gangi A, Guth, S., Imbert, J.P., et al. (2003). Percutaneous vertebroplasty: indications, technique, and results. *Radiographics*, **23**: e10.

Gestin, Y., Vainio, A., Pegurier, A.M. (1997). Long-term intrathecal infusion of morphine in the home care of patients with advanced cancer. *Acta Anaesthesiologica Scandinavica*, **41**: 12–17.

Goetz, M.P., Callstrom, M.R., Charboneau, J.W., et al. (2004). Percutaneous image-guided radiofrequency ablation of painful metastases involving bone: a multicenter study. *Journal of Clinical Oncology*, **22**: 300–306.

Goh, C.R. (2005). Management of incident pain and bone metastases in the palliative care setting. In Justins, D.M., ed. *Pain 2005 – An Updated Review* (Refresher Course Syllabus, 2005), IASP Press, Seattle, 157–169.

Hassenbach, S.J., Cherny, N.I.. Neurosurgical approaches in palliative care. In Doyle, D., Hanks, G., Cherny, N., Calman, K., ed. *Oxford Textbook of Palliative Medicine* (3rd edn) Oxford University Press, Oxford, 396–405.

Hicks, F., Simpson, K.H. (2004). *Nerve Blocks in Palliative Care*. Oxford University Press, Oxford.

Ischia, S., Ischia, A., Luzzani, A., et al. (1985). Results up to death in the treatment of persistent cervico-thoracic (Pancoast) and thoracic malignant pain by unilateral percutaneous cervical cordotomy. *Pain*, **21**: 339–355.

Johnson, M.I., Ashton, C.H., Thompson, J.W. (1991). An in-depth study of long-term users of transcutaneous electrical nerve stimulation (TENS). Implications for clinical use of TENS. *Pain*, **44**: 221–229.

Kaplan, R., Schiff-Keren, B., Alt, E. (1995). Aortic dissection as a complication of celiac plexus block. *Anesthesiology*, **83**: 632–635.

Kanpolat, Y., Savas, A., Ucar, T., Torun, F. (2002). CT-guided percutaneous selective cordotomy for treatment of intractable pain in patients with malignant pleural mesothelioma. *Acta Neurochirurgica*, **144**: 595–599.

Kotani, N., Hashimoto, H., Sato, Y., et al. (2001). Preoperative intradermal acupuncture reduces postoperative pain, nausea and vomiting, analgesic requirement, and sympathoadrenal responses, *Anesthesiology*, **95**: 349–356.

Krainick, J.U., Thoden, U. (1974). Experience with dorsal column stimulation (DCS) in the operative treatment of chronic intractable pain. *Journal of Neurosurgical Sciences*, **18**: 187–189.

Liossi, C. (2000). Clinical hypnosis in paediatric oncology: a critical review of the literature. *Sleep and Hypnosis*, **2**: 125–131.

MacPherson, H., Thomas, K., Walters, S., Fitter, M. (2001). A prospective survey of adverse events and treatment reactions following 34,000 consultations with professional acupuncturists. *Acupuncture in Medicine*, **19**: 93–102.

Malone, B.T., Beye, R., Walker, J. (1985). Management of pain in the terminally ill by administration of epidural narcotics. *Cancer*, **55**: 438–440.

Meglio, M., Cioni, B., Rossi, G.F. (1989). Spinal cord stimulation in the management of chronic pain. A 9–year experience. *Journal of Neurosurgery*, **70**: 519–524.

Miguel, R. (2000). Interventional treatment of cancer pain: the fourth step in the World Health Organization analgesic ladder? *Cancer Control*, **7**: 149–156.

Osenbach, R.K., Harvey, S. (2001). Neuraxial infusion in patients with chronic intractable cancer and noncancer pain. Current Pain and Headache Reports, **5**: 241–249.

Patt, R.B., Cousins, M.J. (1998). Techniques for neurolytic neural blockade. In Cousins, M.J., Bridenbaugh, P.O., ed. *Neural Blockade in Clinical Anaesthesia and Management of Pain* (3rd edn) Lippincott-Raven, Philadelphia, 1007–1061.

Petzke, F., Radbruch, L., Zech, D., *et al.* (1999). Temporal presentation of chronic cancer pain: transitory pains on admission to a multidisciplinary pain clinic. *Journal of Pain and Symptom Management*, **17**: 391–401.

Piquet, C.Y., Mallaret, M.P., Lemoigne, A.H., *et al.* (1998). Respiratory depression following administration of intrathecal bupivacaine to an opioid-dependent patient. *Annals of Pharmacotherapy*, **32**: 653–655.

Portenoy, R.K. (1997). Treatment of temporal variations in chronic cancer pain. *Seminars in Oncology*, **5** (Suppl 16): 7–12.

Rousseff, R.T., Simeonov, S. (2004). Intralesional treatment in painful rib metastases. Palliative Medicine, **18**: 259.

Stannard, C. (2003). Stimulation-induced analgesia in cancer pain management. In Sykes, N., Fallon, M.T., Patt, R.B., ed. *Clinical Pain Management: Cancer Pain*, Edward Arnold, London, 245–251.

Swanwick, M., Haworth, M., Lennard, R.F. (2001). The prevalence of episodic pain in cancer: a survey of hospice patients on admission. *Palliative Medicine*, **15**: 9–18.

Swarm, R.A., Karanikolas, M., Cousins, M.J. (2004). Anaesthetic techniques for pain control. In Doyle, D., Hanks, G., Cherny, N., Calman, K., ed. *Oxford Textbook of Palliative Medicine* (3rd edn) Oxford University Press, Oxford, 378–396.

Thompson, J.W. (1998). Transcutaneous electrical nerve stimulation (TENS). In Filshie, J., White, A., ed. *Medical Acupuncture: A Western Scientific Approach*. Churchill Livingstone, Edinburgh, 177–192.

Twycross, R. (1994). The risks and benefits of corticosteroids in advanced cancer. *Drug Safety*, **11**: 163–178.

Wagemans, M.F., Zuurmond, W.W., de Lange, J.J. (1997). Long-term spinal opioid therapy in terminally ill cancer pain patients. *Oncologist*, **2**: 70–75.

White, A. (1999). Neurophysiology of acupuncture analgesia. In Ernst, E., White, A., ed. *Acupuncture: A Scientific Appraisal*. Butterworth-Heinemann, Oxford, 60–92.

White, A., Hayhoe, S., Hart, A., Ernst, E. (2001). Survey of adverse events following acupuncture (SAFA): a prospective study of 32,000 consultations. *Acupuncture in Medicine*, **19**: 84–92.

Wild, M.R., Espie, C.A. (2004). The efficacy of hypnosis in the reduction of procedural pain and distress in pediatric oncology: a systematic review. *Journal of Developmental and Behavioral Pediatrics*, **25**: 207–213.

Williams, J.E. (2003). Nerve blocks – chemical and neurolytic agents. In Sykes, N., Fallon, M.T., Patt, R.B., ed. *Clinical Pain Management. Cancer Pain*. Oxford University Press, New York, 235–244.

Woolf, C.J., Thompson, J.W. (1994). Stimulation fibre-induced analgesia: transcutaneous electrical nerve stimulation (TENS) and vibration. In Wall, P.D., Melzack, R., ed. *Textbook of Pain* (3rd edn). Churchill Livingstone, New York, 1191–1208.

Yaksh T.L., Malmberg A.B., (1994). Interaction of spinal modulatory receptor systems. In Fields H.L., Liebeskind J.C., ed. *Pharmacological approaches to the treatment of chronic pain: New concepts and critical issues*. IASP Press, Seattle, 151–171.

Zech, D.F., Grond, S., Lynch, J. et al. (1995). Validation of World Health Organization Guidelines for cancer pain relief: a 10–year prospective study. *Pain*, **63**: 65–76.

Zeppetella, G., Ribeiro, M.D. (2003). Pharmacotherapy of cancer-related episodic pain. *Expert Opinion on Pharmacotherapy*, **4**: 493–502.

# Index

111